Heidelberg
Science
Library

Patricia T. Kelly

Dealing with Dilemma

A Manual for Genetic Counselors

Springer-Verlag
New York
Heidelberg
Berlin

Patricia T. Kelly, Ph.D.
G. W. Hooper Foundation
University of California, San Francisco
San Francisco, California 94143

Library of Congress Cataloging in Publication Data

Kelly, Patricia T.   1942–
   Dealing with dilemma.

   (Heidelberg science library)
   Bibliography: p.
   1. Genetic counseling. I. Title. II. Series.
RB155.K44   613.9   77-1803

ISBN 0-387-90237-6 Springer-Verlag New York

ISBN 3-540-90237-6 Springer-Verlag Berlin Heidelberg

To Bernard

Preface

The aim of DEALING WITH DILEMMA is to integrate medical and genetic information with the psychosocial aspects of genetic counseling, in order to provide a working manual for genetic counselors.

The book fills a gap in the genetic counseling field because it emphasizes the humanistic aspects of genetic counseling, and is primarily concerned with communication between genetic counselor and counselee. The few genetic counseling books available at this time are devoted almost entirely to the medical and genetic aspects of the subject.

This book is written in nontechnical language, but it presupposes some knowledge of Mendelian genetics, polygenic inheritance, and chromosomal anomalies. No prior study of psychology or counseling is necessary, however.

DEALING WITH DILEMMA is intended for physician and nonphysician genetic counselors, private practice physicians in pediatrics, obstetrics, family and general practice, internists, nurses, public health professionals, genetic counseling students, social workers, and other health professionals. Much of the material presented should be useful to those who deal with the psychosocial ramifications of many nongenetic diseases as well—problems of the mentally retarded, handicapped, or chronically ill. In addition, it is hoped that professionals who plan state and federal health policy can use this book to gain a better knowledge of the humanistic side of genetic counseling.

For the reader's convenience, there are two Appendices to this volume: Appendix A presents suggested interview schedules and Appendix B is a Glossary of Genetic Diseases for use as a quick reference.

Acknowledgments

I would like to acknowledge the help of A. Russell Lee, M.D., Director of Family Therapy Training, Contra Costa County Mental Health Services, Martinez, California, in the initial organization of much of the material in Chapter 6. I am indebted to him for his perceptive insights and help in conceptualizing many facets of genetic counseling. I would also like to thank Irving K. Zola, Ph.D., Brandeis University, for his creative encouragement, thoughtful suggestions, and patience in reviewing early drafts of this manuscript. Discussions I have had with Alexander G. Rogerson, M.D., Berkeley Pediatric Medical Group, proved extremely valuable in helping me to formulate my thoughts about genetic counseling and the private practitioner. Norma Haan, Ph.D., Director, Genetic Counseling Option, University of California, Berkeley, reviewed several early chapters and encouraged the book's completion. Carol Fegté, Senior Editor, G. W. Hooper Foundation, University of California, San Francisco, has provided much appreciated editorial advice. Lydia Momotuk, Associate Librarian at the University of California, San Francisco, and Carol Yates, Research Assistant at the University of California, Berkeley, greatly aided my search for relevant materials. For their assistance in preparation of the manuscript and typing, many thanks to Claudia Madison and Maureen Morris. Above all, I thank the individuals and families whom I have seen nobly wrestling with their dilemmas in genetic counseling sessions. I hope I have been helpful to them. They may not know it, but they have helped me.

Patricia T. Kelly

Contents

Questions Genetic Counselors Ask   120

Appendix A: Intake and Follow-up Interview Schedules   132

Appendix B: Glossary of Genetic Diseases   137

Bibliography   140

1 Introduction

Exploring these feelings (about the birth of a child with a birth defect) may be far more important than providing a statistical estimate of the risk, and somewhere during the counseling process there should be an opportunity to do so, but in practice this aspect of counseling tends to be neglected.

F. C. Fraser, 1974

Genetic issues are much in the forefront of public concern these days. Newspapers carry reports of new discoveries in the detection of genetic diseases, as well as reports of campaigns to screen various populations for carriers of a genetic disease, particularly Tay-Sachs and sickle cell anemia. Magazine articles ponder the effects of new discoveries on the gene pool, and books such as Etzioni's *Genetic Fix* (1973) debate some of the ethical issues raised by the discovery of such new techniques as amniocentesis, which makes it possible to prenatally determine the sex of unborn children and the presence of genetic defects.

Out of this widespread public awareness and the scientific advances that have been made, there has developed, in little more than a decade, a growing demand for genetic counseling services. In 1957 there were only 13 centers in the United States which formally provided genetic counseling; by 1974 there were over 350 (Hammons, 1959; Bergsma et al., 1974). Their numbers continue to increase, but the need for genetic counseling services at present far exceeds the available supply of trained counselors. Though it is estimated that from 10 to 25 percent of admissions to modern pediatric hospitals are cases of clearly genetic etiology, only a small proportion of the cases receive counseling (Fraser, 1974).

In the early stages of its development, genetic counseling took place mostly on university campuses, sometimes as a voluntary service rendered by a few concerned geneticists. Of the 13 centers existing in 1957, 10 were at universities. Since then, genetic counseling has increasingly become a service offered within a medical rather than a university setting (Sorenson, 1971). Advances in medicine have made pre- and postnatal diagnoses more accurate, so that in establishing a pattern of inheritance, genetic counselors now generally rely more on clinical diagnosis than on pedigree analysis.

Two of genetic counseling's essential elements are genetics and diagnosis. Obviously, without an accurate diagnosis and a thorough knowledge of genetics, accurate genetic counseling cannot occur. The third essential element, communication, has not always been so obvious.

Opinions differ as to how genetic counseling should best be provided. The conventional approach has viewed the genetic counselor's task as the presentation of scientific and medical facts and nothing more. Counseling has generally been structured around a single session, during which the diagnosis has been made or confirmed and the factual information provided, usually by a physician. One visit has usually been considered sufficient. In books or articles that stem from this approach, the counselor has been exhorted to be gentle and compassionate when presenting what is often painful or difficult material to absorb, but this has usually been couched in general terms. Little consideration has been given to trying to determine what specifically might be done to ensure that the compassion manifested by the counselor contributes effectively to the needs of those being counseled. Similarly, it has been an accepted canon of conventional genetic counseling that the process should be "nondirective," but no clarification of this term is to be found and no guidelines are available that outline how the genetic counselor must act in order to achieve or maintain this stance.

The approach set forth in the pages that follow differs from the conventional view. In this book, the essential question is not whether information has been transmitted, but whether it has been understood and assimilated. Different families with the same disease frequently have different concerns and therefore need to learn about different aspects of the disease. The same words may have different meanings to different people, either because their cultural background is different or because they have little familiarity with the medical and genetic terms being used. Effective counselors must recognize these nuances and act accordingly. They know that the people they are counseling must be able to evaluate the significance of the disease and the magnitude of the risk in terms that are meaningful *to them*. To bring about this kind of understanding, the effective genetic counselor must learn how to take information from his or her own frame of reference and transpose it onto the counselee's frame of reference.

Sometimes even that is not enough. Often the threat or suggestion of genetic disease may arouse emotions that create barriers to communication: anxiety, fear, anger, loss of self-esteem, etc. In many genetic counseling situations the emotions are particularly intense because individuals are grieving not just for the present, but for the loss of a healthy future for their present or prospective children. Individuals may not listen to the genetic counselor because they fear they will be given bad news; they may worry so much about their spouses' disapproval of bad genes in the family that they simply no longer hear what is being said to them. Curt Stern (1973) has written, "It is not sufficient to tell the truth; it is necessary to tell the truth humanely." The statement is eloquent, yet it does not go far enough. It has to be recognized that it is not sufficient to tell the truth humanely; it is necessary that the truth be not merely told, but *understood*. Unless counseling skills are used to overcome the barriers to communication (which are often not logical or rational), the counselees will not adequately understand the information being presented no matter how humanely it has been stated.

The view put forth throughout this book is one that is gradually gaining acceptance in principle, though it has not yet been sufficiently translated into practice. In 1975 the Ad Hoc Committee on Genetic Counseling of the American Society of Human Genetics described genetic counseling as "a communication process which deals with the human problems associated with the occurrence, or the risk of occurrence, of a genetic disorder in a family." There is growing agreement, as Fraser's words at the beginning of this chapter attest, that for this communication process to succeed, more is involved than merely a clear statement of the facts.

This book is an outgrowth of my experiences as a genetic counselor and also as a teacher of genetic counseling. As a genetic counselor, it became apparent to me that appropriate counseling techniques were frequently necessary to transmit information to individuals who were having difficulty listening due to their intense emotions, to help individuals voice their unique or special concerns, to present information so that different kinds of people could understand it, and to determine the extent to which people could apply the information to their own lives—that is, whether they had grasped the necessary information to the fullest and most meaningful degree. In teaching genetic counseling, I soon saw that beginning genetic counselors could benefit from a structure around which to build their own counseling practices.

The aim of this book, then, is to show, in an orderly and constructive manner, how to conduct genetic counseling sessions. In presenting genetic counseling as a process consisting of discrete stages, I have sought to provide health professionals with techniques and guidelines for structuring their sessions, and I have sought to explicate for beginning counselors how and when to present genetic information to their clients, how to assess the effectiveness of their genetic counseling, and how to relate genetic counseling to their existing professional skills. Such an approach, I am convinced, enables genetic counselors not merely to transmit accurate information, not merely to convey sympathy, but to deal most usefully with their clients' dilemmas.

To that end, the book is organized essentially as a manual that works through the sequence of processes that the genetic counselor is likely to encounter, considering along the way specific genetic counseling problems that may arise—the anger of a husband who refuses to believe that an albino child can be biologically his offspring; the frustration of a genetic counselor or physician who realizes that the distraught people before him are not really hearing the information he is giving them about the risk of having another Down's child; the anguish of a couple who wishes to have a son but are being told that the probability of a son having Duchenne's muscular dystrophy is 50 percent. Throughout the book, the emphasis is on *normal* reactions to genetic disease that can be handled by practitioners who are perceptive but not necessarily trained in mental health. (A section on how to refer individuals to mental health experts is included.)

Chapter 2 presents a suggested format for genetic counseling in terms of a structured sequence of visits. The various objectives of each visit are briefly described. Throughout this and other chapters, I have quoted liberally from transcripts of counseling sessions I have conducted, taking care, of course, to disguise in each case the identity of the speaker and his or her family. Chapter 3 describes the intake visit—its function, structure, and stages. In Chapter 4, ways of presenting pertinent genetic information are discussed. Chapter 5 contains not only a discussion of how to conduct follow-up visits, but an annotated transcript of a follow-up session. The transcript is intended to give readers a sense of the dynamics of a session; the annotation provides a running commentary by the author on what is happening and what the counselor is seeking to accomplish. Individuals' reactions to genetic disease are presented in Chapter 6 in order to acquaint genetic counselors with the range of responses typically encountered. In Chapter 7, both general and specific genetic counseling techniques are offered, including how to open and close genetic counseling sessions, matters of timing, and various listening skills. The sociologic aspects of genetic counseling are discussed in Chapter 8. This includes such topics as cultural differences in reactions to disease, and communication within medical settings. In Chapter 9, ways of dealing with a wide variety of specific genetic counseling situations are proposed and discussed.

To date, no single term for the people who seek genetic counseling has evolved. In some genetic counseling services, the term "patient" is used. This is not entirely satisfactory, since most of the people counseled are not ill, have no disease, and some are not even known carriers of a genetic disease. The term "client" is sometimes used, but its major drawback is that it reminds one of a lawyer's or psychologist's practice. Increasingly, "counselee" is used, even though it is sometimes confused with "counselor." I use such terms occasionally, but I generally prefer to use such familiar words as "couple," "family," "individual," and "people." Since, after all, even the healthiest of us carries a genetic load of three to five deleterious genes, these more homely terms may help remind us that the counselees *are* people, just like the counselor, even in their genes.

2 Overview of the Genetic Counseling Process

Sickness is a matter of alarm, not of logic. Even when society acts with a logical end in view, it must be prepared to yield at many points to the nonlogical sentiments of the individual whose survival is threatened.

E. D. Churchill, 1949

When genetic counseling is structured around only a single session, as is often the case, or when the service is seen merely as one in which the genetic counselor's main focus and expertise is diagnosis, the counseling aspects of genetic counseling may be overlooked or shortchanged. Obviously, the accuracy of genetic counseling requires accurate diagnosis. What has been less obvious is that for the process to be effective, as well as accurate, sufficient time must be arranged for counseling to take place. The counseling process is one that cannot be forced, skimped, or hurried—not if it is to be meaningful.

Assuming, as I do, therefore, that a sequence of visits is the most desirable format, I am providing in this chapter a general view of how genetic counseling can be organized to facilitate both the diagnostic and counseling aspects of genetic counseling. As shown in Diagram 1, the process is conceived as being divided into four separable stages: preparation, intake visit, diagnostic visit, and follow-up visit. In actual genetic counseling situations, these stages are not always clearly defined. For example, some of the steps listed under preparation may occur during the intake visit, or the diagnostic stage may require several visits that shade into the follow-up stage. However, the stages are presented separately here in order to provide a clear picture of the different processes involved.

Preparation for First Visit

Several steps must occur before the initial visit. First, the individual or family must become aware that there is a genetic problem or a potential genetic problem and must seek genetic counseling, either on their own initiative or their physician's. The persons or families concerned may be referred for genetic counseling by family physicians, specialists (e.g., pediatricians), friends, or family. Increasingly, individuals are referring themselves, after having read of such a service in newspapers or having heard of it on television.

When one talks with people who have come for genetic counseling, one finds expressed a wide variety of motives and expectations. Some are realistic in their concerns. For example, one man who suffered from a hemorrhaging disorder of unknown etiology, gave as his reason for seeking genetic counseling: "Well, I'm hoping that if they can't determine where the bad gene came from, they can at least tell me whether or not my children might have it."*

Some seek genetic counseling because they view it as a new service they feel they ought to take advantage of, now that it has become available. A woman whose grandmother had Huntington's disease said: "Actually I think our feeling right now is that we're doing about as much as we can. And what else can you do?"

Some have a relative with a genetic disease and wish to avoid having a child with the same problem. One woman who wanted to know if she was a carrier for Tay Sachs disease said:

If I'm not a carrier, then it's not important for the prospective father to go through the test. If I am, then it might be a good idea, because I've seen the baby and I've seen my cousins. I know what they're going through. It's really incredible. It's a hard trip.

Some seek genetic counseling as a kind of emotional insurance policy, a way to preclude or assuage future guilt. If, after seeking genetic counseling, they have a child with a birth defect, they feel they will blame themselves less than if they had never sought counseling. One father of a

---

*This man's words, as well as other quotations throughout the book, are from counseling sessions conducted by the author. In each case, of course, care has been taken to disguise the identity of the speaker and his or her family.

DIAGRAM 1: OVERVIEW OF GENETIC COUNSELING PROCESS

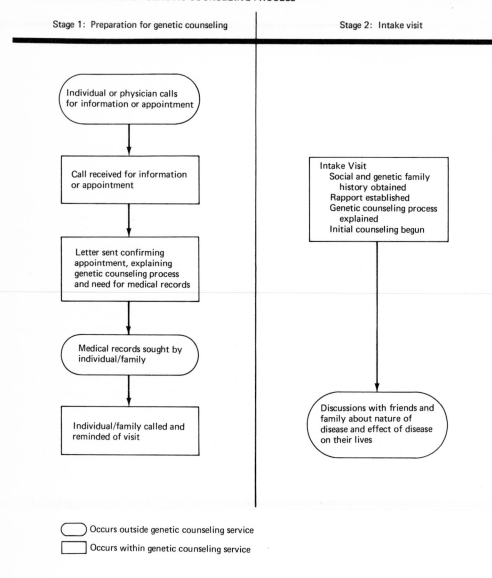

Stage 1: Preparation for genetic counseling | Stage 2: Intake visit

Individual or physician calls for information or appointment

Call received for information or appointment

Letter sent confirming appointment, explaining genetic counseling process and need for medical records

Medical records sought by individual/family

Individual/family called and reminded of visit

Intake Visit
   Social and genetic family
      history obtained
   Rapport established
   Genetic counseling process
      explained
   Initial counseling begun

Discussions with friends and family about nature of disease and effect of disease on their lives

Occurs outside genetic counseling service
Occurs within genetic counseling service

Stage 3: Diagnostic visit(s)   Stage 4: Follow-up visit(s)

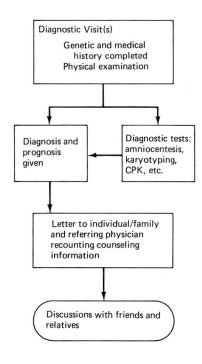

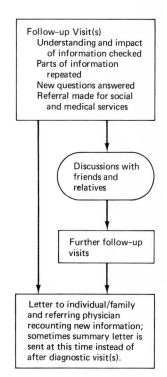

Down's syndrome child put it: "So we just want to do all we can and not say 10 or 15 years from now what we should have done at this time."

Others come to the center with vague, even unrealistic or confused notions about what genetic counseling may offer them. One woman, whose daughter has Pierre Robin syndrome, asked: "Can't the geneticists look inside your chromosomes and check to see if there's any possibility of you carrying a bad gene?"

Individuals may make the decision to seek genetic counseling just after learning for the first time that there is a potential genetic problem (e.g., immediately following the birth of a child with hydrocephalus), or many years after the disorder is recognized (e.g., a woman whose brother has Duchenne's muscular dystrophy). Starting with the initial telephone contact, the genetic counselor should explain in general terms how the genetic service is structured, including the usual number and timing of visits. If there is a referring physician, the genetic counselor should speak with him or her to learn more about the client's needs, as well as aspects of the case that are of special interest or concern to the referring doctor.

Many individuals who call for genetic counseling naturally feel sensitive about their medical problem (see Chapter 6). Thus, tact should be exercised by the genetic counselor or clinic staff during this initial telephone call. Such terms as "deformity," "defect," or "abnormality" should be avoided during these discussions. Some people may need the reassurance of several telephone conversations with the genetic service before they follow through with their initial visit.

Following the initial telephone conversation, it is useful for the staff to confirm the appointment with the family in writing and to reiterate directions, projected timing and number of visits, family members expected to participate, and the need for various medical records. By asking individuals to begin the collection of pertinent medical records before the initial or intake visit, much time can be saved. Staff members should be specific when requesting records, since individuals without experience in medical matters may view this request as a call for all records from a large number of extended family members, and spend considerable time obtaining material that will be of little use.

Intake Visit The intake visit is usually the first face-to-face meeting of family and genetic counseling personnel, and does much to determine the tone of subsequent genetic counseling visits.

During this session rapport is established and information exchanged. Usually both spouses, but not small children, attend this visit. The genetic counseling service should provide child care for parents who need it. If child care is not possible, appropriate playthings should be provided for the children so parents are not distracted.

During the intake visit, the genetic counselor provides detailed information about procedures to be followed and those personnel who will be involved in the genetic counseling process. For example, if the counselor suspects that the family's child has Turner's syndrome, the counselor should tell the parents that during the next visit blood will probably be drawn from the child and a karyotype analysis will be performed by trained technicians. In addition, parents need to be assured that there will be time for discussion of the test results. During this visit the genetic counselor should also provide appropriate background information about genetics and medicine (e.g., definition of chromosomes or karyotype analysis).

For many people, an overview of what to expect can help alleviate the anxiety that they may feel in a new situation, particularly in a clinic or hospital setting. As one man said:

> Hospitals, doctors, clinics, all frighten most of us, or intimidate us, anyway. I feel intimidated whenever I walk into a hospital, even if I'm a visitor. You smell those nasty smells and see those straight-faced people.

Appropriate background information about genetics and medicine is useful to most people, because it helps them to begin formulating their concerns in a way that can be answered by the genetic counselor. One woman, whose two children had congenital cataracts, initially said:

> I only wish I had more questions to ask. You know, intelligible questions pertaining to the children. After all these years you would think I would have something more, but it's like stabbing in the dark.

Since many people are unsure what genetic counseling involves, a genetic counselor can help by telling them what the service does and does not include. Counselees may need to realize that genetic counseling has its limits. For example, one man said: "What we're looking for is whether or not we check out as normal." It is important to correct such misconceptions early, so that the client can devote his or her energies to learning what realistically can be accomplished through genetic counseling.

During the intake visit information is obtained from the family not only about medical and genetic aspects of their problem, but also relevant social aspects, including the impact of the disease on their lives, and the family's particular questions and concerns. During this visit the genetic counselor learns how the family views and defines the problem. It is at this point that the counselor can help the family define what it wants and what it can get from the genetic counseling service. Such an early understanding of individuals' concerns can help genetic counselors later present information in a way that the family can best understand and use.

In addition to providing information, the intake visit can show individuals that the genetic counselor or clinic is willing to provide emotional support and to listen to their individual concerns. Such an understanding often makes it possible for individuals to speak of their concerns and ask questions without embarrassment or fear of being judged stupid or incompetent. One woman who was diagnosed as an epileptic said about her intake visit: "What we got was that you're really interested in dealing with people and helping them with what their needs are and straightening out any miscommunication."

Diagnostic Visit   The diagnostic visit comes next. Usually a wait of about a week between intake and diagnostic visits is advisable, but if medical records are not available or long distances must be traveled, the time between visits may be lengthened or shortened. Spacing the visits gives individuals an opportunity to digest and synthesize the information they have received during the intake visit, to contact relatives, and to continue discussions about the disease and genetic counseling within the family. Frequently individuals report that because discussions started during the intake visit are continued at home, greater mutual understanding and support occur within the family so that they are able to approach the diagnostic visit in a more informed and focused manner than before the intake visit. Instead of waiting for the genetic counselor to tell them what they should know, they now have questions to ask the counselor.

If a pedigree has not been taken or completed during the intake visit, it should be done during the diagnostic visit.

Physical examinations are also given to make or confirm the diagnosis. As a consequence of information obtained from the pedigree and/or the physical examinations, further medical records from relatives may be needed. Various laboratory tests and procedures may be ordered, for example karyotyping of blood or skin, amniocentesis, or a CPK test to determine carrier status for muscular dystrophy. In some cases the consultation of a pathologist, neurologist, hematologist, or other type of medical specialist is indicated. Several diagnostic visits may be needed before all the available information is obtained and it is determined whether a diagnosis can be made.

Once the diagnosis is established (or it becomes apparent that the diagnosis cannot be established with certainty at this time), the direct informational aspects of genetic counseling can begin. While waiting for the diagnosis to be established, the counselor either gives no diagnostic information ("I know it is hard to wait, but we won't know what the risk to future children is until the tests are completed and we have more concrete information about what the problem is."), or gives such information only in couched terms ("Well, it looks like Ehlers-Danlos syndrome, but we can't be completely sure until all the tests are completed."). Once the diagnosis is established, the counselor explains how it was determined, and its implications for present and future children.

Follow-up Visits Follow-up visits usually occur one to three weeks after the diagnostic visit, but may be scheduled earlier to meet specific individual or family needs. Generally, it helps to have some time between visits, so that individuals can discuss the findings of the diagnostic visit with friends and relatives and begin integrating the information they have received into their lives and value systems. Often new questions arise as a result of this integration. Also, friends and relatives frequently ask questions that the individuals did not think to ask during the diagnostic visit. Follow-up visits provide a time for such questions to be answered.

Since much genetic counseling information is technical, the information often has to be repeated several times before individuals can grasp it. Follow-up visits enable the genetic counselor to ascertain whether the information has been correctly understood and assessed. These follow-up visits also allow the counselor to deal with the denial or distortion of information that may occur when the individual is under the emotional strain of having to deal with painful or unwelcome data (see Chapter 5). Even when the genetic counseling information is of a welcome nature, individuals may have a difficult time understanding or accepting it. For example, one woman with oculocutaneous albinism (who is quoted at length in Chapter 5) said:

> I got out of it [genetic counseling] that I shouldn't worry about it. That the incidence in the population is extremely low and the probability that Henry would have a recessive gene that would produce an albino baby is *really* low, and I shouldn't even be concerned about worrying about it. *However,* I've been used to worrying about it for so long, I'm not sure it's that easy to just stop it and erase it.

An essential part of genetic counseling is the referral of individuals to appropriate social services. Follow-up visits provide the best opportunity to make such referrals. For example, a couple with a Down's baby may need to learn that it is possible to enroll their child in an Early Infant Stimulation Program. Though such services may be mentioned in the diagnostic visit, their implementation should occur during a follow-up visit. Since follow-up visits are for discussion and planning, parents should be encouraged to leave young children at home or in the genetic counseling service's child care facility.

Follow-up Letter   An important, even essential, element of follow-up is a letter to both the individual and the referring physician. It should not be a form letter. It should recount the primary questions clients had and provide whatever information is available to answer these questions (including diagnosis, type of inheritance, risk figures and how these were derived). If the letter is sent subsequent to follow-up visits, it should also include a summary of the follow-up visits, including the names and addresses of relevant specialists and social services. Technical language should be avoided when possible in this letter. When technical terms must be used, they should be defined, even if clients seemed to understand them during counseling. For example, the genetic counselor might write, "As you remember, we talked about amniocentesis. In this procedure, a small amount of fluid is. . . ." Such definitions ensure that individuals will not become confused when the letter is reread long after genetic counseling has been completed. Also, many people use such a letter to explain to friends and relatives the information they have received and to refresh their own memory as time goes by. In some cases the letter serves to reassure people that they indeed heard the information correctly. In this letter it is important that the basic concerns clients expressed during genetic counseling be addressed and that they be encouraged to call or write if the information is not complete, or if more information is desired at a future time.

Whenever possible, it is useful for the staff member who conducted the intake visit to be present during the family's diagnostic and follow-up visits as well. Not only do families report that they feel more at ease during a diagnostic visit if a familiar staff person is with them, but the staff member can ensure that issues of concern are clearly brought to the diagnostician's attention during the diagnostic visit. During follow-up visits, the staff member who has followed the family through the genetic counseling process can check to see that initial concerns and questions were answered, and that the genetic counseling information is being understood.

3 Intake Visit

The patient does not know what he is supposed to do nor in any clear way what he wants or expects the doctor to do.

I. K. Zola, 1964

The intake visit is usually the first face-to-face meeting between the family and the genetic counselor or clinic member. As such, this visit sets the stage for future interaction between the family and the genetic counseling service, and can do much to develop the trust and open communication necessary for effective genetic counseling. Depending on the structure of the genetic counseling service, the intake visit may be conducted by a geneticist, physician, master of genetic counseling, social worker, or nurse. Regardless of who collects initial information (social, genetic, medical), it is important that the intake interviewer maintain contact with the family throughout the genetic counseling process and communicate relevant information to other staff members.

A major aim of the intake visit, as has been noted, is to establish rapport with family members. The establishment of rapport is crucial. With rapport established, it becomes possible for the family to voice their concerns freely, to ask the questions that need to be asked and to pay heed to the answers given, to admit frankly when they have failed to understand, and to examine their own often turbulent emotions honestly. In short, it becomes possible for communication to take place. Without rapport, a counseling session is doomed to failure. Under these circumstances even the best-presented genetic counseling information may not be believed by the family. Their reaction may be to refuse to admit that a genetic problem exists, despite the evidence offered them. Or, lacking confidence in that particular genetic counseling service, they may go shopping around for other medical advice or, as some do, seek miraculous solutions from faith healers.

During a successful intake visit, information will not only pass from family to genetic counselor, but from counselor to family as well. At the end of the intake visit, both should have a better understanding of each other and what the genetic counseling process will involve in this case. Generally, this understanding will be achieved if the genetic counselor:

1. Provides the family with information about genetic counseling procedures and personnel;
2. Explores the medical and genetic aspects of the disease;
3. Explores the social aspects and impact of the disease;
4. Prepares the family for the diagnostic visit—factually;
5. Prepares the family for the diagnostic visit—emotionally.

Providing the Family with Information about Genetic Counseling Procedures and Personnel

In seeking genetic counseling, most individuals do not know what to expect. Not only is genetic counseling a relatively new field, but, as at least one study suggests, laymen do not have either specific or firmly held expectations about the services or specialists they desire in a health setting (Lipton and Svarstad, 1974). Therefore, whether seeking counseling from either a team or a single physician, individuals wonder: Will they have to undress? How many people will examine them? Will blood be drawn? What tests will be done? Will they be seen by a physician or by a geneticist? How much time (in weeks or months) will the genetic counseling take? Parents wonder if they will have an opportunity to consult with the genetic counselor out of their children's hearing, what facilities will be available for their children while they talk to the genetic counselor, and whether the staff will be sympathetic to the needs of their children. They wonder if the genetic counselor will be someone of whom they can ask questions without feeling stupid, and whom they can trust. As one father whose daughter had tuberous sclerosis said: "When you talk with somebody about something like that, you feel like you've got to have some kind of trust there first." One way to establish trust is to give families a general understanding of what the genetic counseling process is likely to involve and the structure of the particular counseling service. A discussion of the counseling structure should always include information on fees. When it is not possible to be exact about them, the genetic counselor should give the family an estimate of the total cost, noting the areas of uncertainty. The family's ability to pay for counseling can be determined, and a payment schedule devised. If the family does not feel comfortable with the fee, they may not complete counseling, or may enter into counseling with nagging worries about their finances. Financial worries can keep people from voicing their needs and concerns, for example, a special nursery school for a Down's child. For fear that they may not be able to affort it, parents may insist that their child does not need such care. Therefore, the financial aspects of genetic counseling should be dealt with early in the intake visit.

Individuals seeking counseling are usually curious about the training and qualifications of the genetic counseling staff, as well as its size. A discussion of these topics during the intake visit can help families feel more at ease. Usually it is not necessary to discuss the qualifications of the clinic or staff at great length. Instead, comments about individuals who will be most closely associated with the family can do much to relieve anxiety, for example, "He likes children very much and is quite gentle with them," or "She has been on the staff for two years now, and previously studied with an outstanding geneticist." There is some indication (Reader et al., 1957) that individuals will hesitate to raise issues that are of importance to them in a medical setting. Therefore, the genetic counselor must be prepared to raise issues and encourage the family to do so as well.

Conversations about the staff generally lead to questions about the genetic counseling service itself. People wonder if they have come to the right place for counseling about their disease, if the counselor or clinic has seen cases like theirs before, or is aware of recent research developments pertaining to their disease. Again, simple statements about the counselor's experience or expertise can serve to reduce anxiety, for example, "We see at least five families a year with a child who has Duchenne's muscular dystrophy." Many families also want to be sure that they will be notified if discoveries are made about the disease that concerns them. Often genetic counselors keep a file on families by syndrome so that new information can be easily disseminated. If such a file is maintained, counselees should be told of it.

When genetic counseling occurs in a clinic, there may be aspects of clinic operation that seem strange to a layperson: for example, the clinic conference at which a child or family is presented to a group of specialists. Most families have no objection to participating in a clinic conference if it is explained beforehand that the conference is held to stimulate an exchange of information and ideas about how to deal with the family's problem.

Exploring the Medical and Genetic Aspects of the Disease

During the intake visit, the genetic counselor learns the details of the family's experiences with the disease in question, and takes a family history to determine if there are relatives who might be affected or whose medical records would be useful in making or verifying the diagnosis. It is not unusual for individuals to be reluctant about asking relatives for medical records. Individuals may not want to acknowledge that there might be a genetic or family disease; they may fear such a request will strain relationships with relatives, or they may worry about hurting their relatives' feelings. One woman waited over three months before asking her mother for her mentally retarded brother's records: "And here I am saying, 'Hey, Mom, would you send Bill's records over so I can find out if my kid's gonna be as horrible as yours was.' That's sort of what I felt like I was saying to her." People feel far more justified in asking for records if the genetic counselor takes the time to carefully explain why the records are necessary. In some cases, families may want the counselor to ask their relatives for medical records directly. Sometimes the relatives will also want genetic counseling.

Even if individuals feel no embarrassment in asking relatives for medical records, obtaining them often takes time. By making use of medical and genetic information received during the intake visit (e.g., the need for relatives' medical records or tests for affected family members), the genetic counselor will avoid scheduling premature diagnostic counseling sessions. Not only will the counselor's and the family's time be saved, but rapport with the family will be increased when concern for their time is shown. One man with Alport's syndrome stated: "I don't mind return visits. The thing that ticks me off is a return visit when it's just at the whim of a doctor who didn't bother to ask for the information in the first place."

Exploring the Social Aspects and Impact of the Disease

During the initial visit, clients are often unsure about the propriety of raising, or the way in which to raise, areas that are of concern to them. However, if these same issues are not discussed during genetic counseling, the genetic counselor is often criticized later for "not really caring" about them or not being intelligent enough to realize that these areas are important. The result is that families who do not have an opportunity to discuss areas of concern often listen less ("At a certain point I'm sure I stopped hearing because I was so upset."), learn less, and are therefore less prepared to make their own decisions.

In one family, a mother evinced distress about her mentally retarded daughter's rash. During the intake visit, she spent much of her time talking about remedies she had tried for the rash, as well as complaining about previous physicians and their lack of concern about her daughter. A pediatrician was alerted to the mother's anxieties about the rash and during the diagnostic visit spent some time discussing its nature, occurrence, and possible care. Following this discussion the mother stopped concentrating on the rash, stopped berating doctors, and began asking substantial questions about her daughter's mental retardation. Her husband subsequently commented:

> I think that it was really great that we were able to see you ahead of time so that you would know something about us and what our hangups might be. It wasn't just an all of a sudden coming together with a doctor without any knowledge or background.

Sometimes the initial visit will reveal that spouses disagree about the severity of a disease or its consequences to future children. These disagreements are sometimes not openly acknowledged until a later session or are presented as being of little consequence. When disagreements are not discussed and explored during the initial interview, open genetic counseling is often difficult to achieve. Because of the disagreements, spouses are reluctant to bring up topics or questions for fear of starting discussions which will involve "touchy issues." When spouses disagree, the genetic counselor can do much to pave the way for open discussions by establishing a nonjudgmental tone during the initial interview. (Specific techniques for dealing with disagreements are given in Chapter 9.) When a team is involved in counseling, alerting other members of the team to the disagreement will, of course, help them present information and counseling judiciously.

The intake visit also enables the genetic counselor to start becoming aware of the social and emotional impact of the disease on the family unit. Such knowledge helps the genetic counselor judge the speed at which information can be assimilated by the family, as well as areas of information which may have to be repeated or stressed to ensure comprehension. For example, a couple who had a child with Potter's syndrome were shocked that a baby of theirs could look so grotesque. Careful probing by the genetic counselor revealed that this couple was most upset by the abnormal positioning of the hands and feet. In subsequent discussions, the counselor carefully explained that the failure of the kidneys to develop resulted in a lack of amniotic fluid during fetal life, which in turn led to fetal compression and consequent abnormal positioning of hands and feet. If the counselor had not understood this couple's major concern about the hands and feet, this aspect of fetal development might not have been as thoroughly discussed.

A knowledge of the social impact of the disease is essential if the genetic counselor is to understand the *family's* definition of the disease, its seriousness, and consequences to other family members. For example, a woman whose brother has hemophilia and is frequently hospitalized will have different feelings about the disease than a woman who has only sisters. These two women may therefore have completely different reactions when they learn that they are carriers for hemophilia. Sometimes clients worry that their reactions to genetic disease are extreme or abnormal, when in fact they are quite normal, e.g., grief and anger. These people are frequently helped by being told what some of the normal responses are.

In addition to genetic diseases, individuals should be asked about any serious or prolonged illness in themselves or their family. People frequently extrapolate from one disease to another. Therefore, the genetic counselor needs to point out that the medical and social effects of one disease are not necessarily the same as another.

Preparing the Family for the Diagnostic Stage— Factually

Terms and concepts used in genetic counseling are often technical and specialized. Yet to understand their disease or the options available to them, families must acquire some knowledge of genetics, statistics, embryology, and biochemistry, along with the appropriate vocabulary. The intake visit provides a time to help individuals gain the knowledge needed to make an informed decision. One woman, who had come to see whether she was a translocation carrier, said about her intake visit:

> I think once we came here and discussed it with you, it really made it easy to come in. We had our thoughts lined up as to what was expected instead of going in cold. You really have *no* idea. It's hard for you to understand, but people don't have the vaguest idea of what a chromosome study is. It (an explanation of the test) alleviates the fears of walking in the front door.

Much of genetic counseling revolves around questions of risk and probability. Many people appear to be knowledgeable about such concepts. However few can readily grasp the meaning of a given risk figure as applied to their own lives. One woman thought a 50 percent risk represented "good odds." Subsequent discussion revealed that she thought 50 percent guaranteed her a healthy baby. Education about the meaning of probability and risk can be started during the intake interview. During the intake interview the couple does not usually reach a decision about the risk they would take, nor is a firm risk figure given at this time since the diagnosis has not been made or confirmed. However, counselees are encouraged to begin considering what an acceptable risk would be. It is not only the mathematically unsophisticated who benefit from discussions of risk. One man, a mathematics professor, said:

> Somebody tells you that there's a very slight probability of something disastrous happening. Do you risk it? What are the cut-off points? Is 98 percent good and 96 percent bad? How do you make that kind of decision? It's very hard.

By encouraging people to talk about the uncertainties they face, including the frustrations of dealing with these uncertainties, individuals get an opportunity to learn more about their feelings concerning various risks, given the particular disease and their personal history.

During the intake visit, people often need to learn what they can realistically expect from genetic counseling. Some people are surprised to learn that counseling information is usually given in the form of probabilities. Others hope for a cure resulting from a recent scientific breakthrough. Still others say they have come for "a complete genetic checkup." Some requests are quite poignant: "The baby was born very badly deformed and died almost immediately. We would just like to find out if we could have another child." This woman, like many others, hoped that a genetic counselor would tell her that her genes were all right and thus *guarantee* that the next child would be normal. In this case the medical records and autopsy report were not sufficient for a diagnosis to be made. The couple elected to have amniocentesis during the next pregnancy to rule out a chromosomal disorder. They were initially quite reluctant to believe that there exists no battery of biochemical tests that could be done "to rule out as many genetic diseases as possible." When families are told that an expected test or procedure is either not possible or not useful, they often experience a period of disappointment or even disbelief. They may wonder if the test could be done by a different physician or genetic counseling group. In most cases, education and discussion reassure people that the test cannot be done anywhere. Ideally, by the time of the diagnostic visit, many individuals have a better idea of the types of information genetic counseling can and cannot provide, and so are less likely to be coping with a fresh disappointment during this informational visit.

Preparing the Family for the Diagnostic Stage— Emotionally

Often families who come for genetic counseling have had painful experiences as a result of their disease, and little opportunity to discuss these experiences or their feelings about them. For some, discussion of the problem during the intake visit is the first opportunity they have had to explore the topic in depth. One woman, in whose husband's family Huntington's disease was suspected, commented: "The illnesses that happen in his family aren't discussed. Tragedies like that aren't talked about in any family. It's always hushed. Everyone has fears. Yet no one ever talks about it." Discussions about hitherto hushed diseases can change an individual's views or present alternative views that had not been previously perceived.

Many people report a growing feeling of isolation following the discovery of a genetic disease (see Chapter 6), making communication with others even more difficult. When a genetic problem is visible (e.g., a large head) parents may isolate themselves to avoid embarrassing looks and questions from strangers. Often, friends and relatives are either given incomplete or no information about the problem. For example, one family had a stillborn baby with multiple malformations, including heart defects. Friends and relatives were told only that "the baby had a bad heart." The parents then found themselves with no one to talk to about the other malformations, some of which they found grotesque and frightening. Some individuals report that friends and relatives avoid them out of fear that the disease is contagious and that other pregnant women will catch it.

In some cases, friends and relatives feel that the affected family's troubles and pain will be intensified if the situation is discussed. Individuals' attempts to talk about their fears, feelings of pain, doubts, etc., are therefore rebuffed. One young mother of a Down's child said:

> I haven't talked very much about it. I try to talk to my sister, but she tries to avoid the idea too that he's like that. She says, "Well, don't talk about it. Don't think about it. You'll only hurt yourself." And with my mother it's the same thing. She says, "No, no, just have faith in God." So there isn't anybody to talk to.

When individuals have not had an opportunity to talk about their genetic problems, they often need to fully explain their experiences to the genetic counselor. Some families seem to gain a greater understanding of the effects of the disease on their lives during the retelling. Others express relief that they have been able to "get it off my chest" by talking to the counselor. Still others are convinced that the genetic counselor cannot really understand the disease until he or she has heard the details of the family's experiences with it. Naturally, the degree to which counselees wish to speak about their experiences with the disease varies with the disease and the people. The intake visit, by providing time for people to discuss the social impact of the disease, enables the genetic counselor to better understand what help and information they need. Generally, information transfer is enhanced when family members have been able to speak about their emotional concerns, since:

1. people who are expending energy on supression of emotion cannot give full attention to the information being presented;
2. people need to see how they "feel" about information before the information has relevance;

3. people often gain a greater understanding of their thoughts, feelings, and emotional tolerance in the face of genetic disease by expressing how they feel about their genetic problems.

In summary, the intake interview can do much to meet the need for expressing emotion, and thus prepare people for the more informational aspects of genetic counseling that occur during the diagnostic stage.

4 Diagnostic Visit

The health professional is always in danger of extending his
authority in technical matters over the patient's system of beliefs and
values.

E. D. Pellegrino, 1975

The purpose of the diagnostic visit is to examine family
members, order various diagnostic tests, and inform individuals what diagnosis the physical examinations and tests
indicate. During this visit specialists may be called in or
the decision may be made to consult specialists at a future
time, if necessary.

This chapter does not explain how a genetic counseling
service makes a diagnosis, as that is outside the province
of this book, but will be concerned, rather, with how
information about the diagnosis can best be communicated
to the clients. Too often, in diagnostic settings, the emphasis is placed on the diagnosis and the physician's understanding of the diagnosis, with relatively little attention
paid to the client and the client's understanding of the
diagnosis. The premise of this book, as stressed throughout, is that it is not sufficient to make and present an
accurate diagnosis; fully as important is that the diagnosis
be understood and assimilated by those it affects. It
becomes an essential part of the genetic counselor's job,
therefore, to do whatever is necessary to assure that successful communication takes place. It may require many
repetitions of the information. It may require thoughtful
discussion of issues that might seem medically peripheral
to the counselor but are obviously of pressing concern to

the family. It may require long silences while counselees struggle with their emotions or strive to grasp what they have been told. It may require the marshalling of alternative ways of presenting the technical information. As the perceptive genetic counselor knows, the particular approach to be taken will vary considerably from case to case. However, certain elements are basic to successful communication in genetic counseling and some of these are the subject of this chapter.

The Setting   Obviously, the environment or setting of the diagnostic visit will affect a family's receptivity to diagnostic information. For example, a couple whose baby has just died will find it difficult to concentrate on information if babies are crying in a nearby room. This statement might seem self-evident, yet the frequent inclusion of genetic counseling in pediatric departments too often results in a sharing of space that includes crying infants. A clinical setting (e.g., examining room) also intimidates many people, as one couple observed:

GEORGE: Well, the other thing is the little treatment room.

WENDY: Oh, yes. That was hardly conducive to conversation.

GEORGE: A little teeny room in the clinic building. The clinic building is so bleak, you know. And when you're sitting in a little treatment room that's freezing cold, and you're sort of down under this oppressive situation and a couple of doctors come in and hunch around the treatment table and kind of overwhelm you. You aren't in a position to discuss the gray areas of your case, and so it's boom, boom, you're done.

Therefore, whenever possible, it is best to examine individuals in an examining room, and to hold discussions in another room with easy chairs and a less clinical atmosphere.

Timing   Timing and tact are extremely important in giving information about genetic diseases. Care should be taken not to rush this process. For example, if a diagnosis is strongly suspected but tests are still needed (e.g., for neurofibromatosis), the genetic counselor can give people time to hope and adjust by saying, "Neurofibromatosis is a possibility, but we won't be sure until the tests are in." Too often, in the name of honesty, individuals are not told the diagnosis until it is definite. They are then given this diagnosis in such firm and unequivocal language that there is little time to become accustomed to it. A man with Alport's syndrome summarized what many people have said they feel when they receive new, surprising, or unwelcome information.

> The doctors don't realize the patient is a person and you don't just blurt out scientific facts and figures to him without having some feeling for how he's going to react to it.

In another case a mother reported what happened when she went for a diagnosis about her son's failing eyesight:

> And the news he gave us! I think he used very poor taste. But this was just his way of laying it all out in the clear. He said, "I would not give you any hope that Bruce will see again. His chances of being blind are rather great. You should prepare yourself for the worst." Well, I left there in tears, just panic-stricken, and projected every ounce of fear of blindness that I had onto him over the next two to three weeks.

The child has congenital cataracts, and six years after the reported doctor's visit, wears thick glasses, but can see. At the time of the visit to the doctor, his sight had failed somewhat, but he was still able to see. How much easier for this mother it would have been if the physician had said, "Well, we know that Bruce is going to have some trouble with his sight, but we don't know how much. Let's see what happens. We have a good group of physicians here who will do all that is medically possible to help him."

The mother of a child with Pierre Robin syndrome was given "genetic counseling" shortly after she gave birth. The father said about that experience:

> In that half hour after birth, she needed more comfort than information. He should have let her recover before saying, "All right, this might happen, that might happen." You know, it was like sticking a hypodermic syringe deeper and deeper and saying, "Hey, has that hit you yet?"

Generally, people understand new information best if it is presented in a slow and logical fashion. However, individuals often have pressing questions that they want answered first. If these questions are put off until later, counselees may find it difficult to concentrate fully on the information being presented. Therefore, it is usually worthwhile to elicit questions before starting an explanation. Such questions can give the genetic counselor clues about what concern is uppermost in the individual's mind that day, as well as the language best suited for the explanation. The process works best when information is presented as a sequence, with the counselor making sure that one point is understood before proceeding to the next point (e.g., the formation of germ cells containing half of an individual's genetic material; conception as the bringing together of the two halves to make a whole). Often people will say they understand even if they don't. Such phrases as, "Is that making sense?"; "I'm not sure that was easy to follow."; "Perhaps I should go over that again?"; give individuals an opportunity to hear small parts of the information again without them having to admit, "I didn't understand most of what you said in the last five minutes."

In describing genetic and medical processes, the counselor should strive to use common terms rather than esoteric ones whenever possible. The individuals with whom he or she is dealing are being asked to absorb on short notice a whole new field of knowledge, and perhaps even a new way of viewing body processes. Technical terms can impede this understanding since people often feel ignorant when they don't know a technical term, and can spend a great deal of time trying to remember a term at the expense of the broader concept. For example, "division" can be used instead of "meiosis," "leg" instead of "tibia," "failure to separate" instead of "nondisjunction." When it is important for individuals to know a technical term, it should be slowly and carefully defined.

Very intelligent people may have little medical or genetic background. Therefore, it is not talking down or being patronizing to use simple terms or to carefully define more difficult terms if they must be used. Such phrases as, "Since it is known that . . .", "Scientists have shown that . . .", and "As you know . . ." can be used to introduce basic information. Generally, people are not affronted by hearing something they know presented clearly and logically. They *are* upset by rushed explanations that don't fully answer their questions and that leave them feeling uninformed and confused.

Tact While it is often important to discuss an individual's appearance and disorder with colleagues, the choice of terms describing the problem should be circumspect when the individual or family is present. Many individuals are sensitive about their medical problem (or assumed medical problem), and react quite negatively to terms such as "defect," "anomaly," "deformity," "abnormality," and "birth defect."

A man with congenital icthyosis said of his visit to a genetics clinic, "I felt like a god-damned animal in a zoo being observed." The mother of a child who was being seen for suspected Turner's syndrome was upset about the way her child was treated and the lack of consideration shown to her and her husband during a clinic conference:

> Well, I was just really upset about the time we came in to see you all. The doctor pulled up her dress and said, "Look at the dent in her chest," took off her shoe, said, "Look at her toe. Look at her feet. See here on her ears?" We hadn't been told what was going to be done. Nobody said that the symptoms were going to be shown to everyone like that.

Her husband was upset for a different reason: "I knew that we were going in there, but I expected a statement as to what kinds of things they had found . . . somehow an involvement of the parents. But there was no involvement." As this father's comment demonstrates, individuals want to feel a part of the counseling process all the way through. Therefore, when tests and further examinations are indicated, the genetic counselor should explain the rationale for them, as well as why they will take time. Such explanations often prevent misunderstandings, as illustrated by this mother who was given an opportunity to ask questions and felt comfortable about asking them:

> He asked if we had any questions, and I asked him about the long-term effects of Turner's syndrome. I asked him about the chromosome test—exactly what was going to be done and what they expected to find out. I asked why it was going to take so *long*. I considered four to six weeks a long time, never considering that it would take even longer.

Concern for the Client in the Organization of Routines

Genetic counselors should try to ensure that they are on time for scheduled appointments and that their appointments are sufficiently spaced so that counselees do not spend long periods of time waiting for the genetic counselor to complete their diagnoses. When people are forced to endure unreasonably long waits they may feel devalued and insignificant to such an extent that they may tune out the genetic information being offered. For example, one father whose daughter had retinitis pigmentosa said:

> Well, the wait was considerable too. We met the doctor, he left, we met him again, and that was to complete what he started on the first go around. Then it was a two or three hour wait and he led us to believe he would be back in half an hour. He did give us the time element, so we didn't go anywhere, like to get a cup of coffee or anywhere else.

During the diagnostic visit, under the pressures of analyzing clinical symptoms and making a diagnosis, it can be difficult for the diagnostician to demonstrate concern for the individual. For example, in one instance a physician was intently asking a woman about the swelling in her joints. The woman seemed to be feeling uncomfortable about her disfiguring condition and the pointed questions asked about it. She began to talk about her capabilities as an artist. She said, ''You might not think it, but even with these hands I can do very good water colors. I had my work in several shows and. . . .'' The physician brushed aside her comments and continued asking for clinical and physical information in order to make a diagnosis. The woman became hostile and was not informative in talking about her physical symptoms.

Because there is often much medical information to be obtained, and making a diagnosis can be difficult and absorbing, the social or human aspects of a disease can sometimes be overlooked. Wolfensberger (1965) cites several examples of diagnostic tools being used to obtain information of interest to the diagnostician, but of relatively little interest to the person with the disease. If a health professional who has a primary commitment to the counseling aspects of genetic counseling (e.g., a Master's in genetic counseling) maintains contact with individuals during the diagnostic visit, many such oversights can be avoided. Alternatively, physicians and geneticists can schedule times for counseling and discussion.

Modes of Inheritance and Chromosomal Disorders   In the following sections are some generalizations on communicating about diseases with different modes of inheritance, uncertain modes of inheritance, and those due to chromosomal disorders. Probability is an integral part of all these explanations, so a separate section is devoted to this topic as well. In all these communications, audiovisual aids can be a great help. Some genetic counselors use films to provide background information to groups with similar problems and in individual counseling sessions as well. Where resources are more limited, simple diagrams have been successfully used, with individuals taking them home for further discussions with friends and relatives.

Chromosomal Disorders

The most frequently encountered chromosomal disorder is, of course, simple trisomy 21, or Down's syndrome. Other chromosome anomalies include Turner's syndrome (XO), Klinefelter's syndrome (XXY), the XYY syndrome, and translocation Down's syndrome. All of these chromosomal disorders are due to either the presence of an extra chromosome (simple trisomy 21), the absence of a chromosome (Turner's syndrome), or a chromosomal rearrangement resulting in either duplication or deletion of genetic material. The family usually comes for genetic counseling following the birth of an affected child. However, individuals occasionally come for genetic counseling before the birth of an affected child to see if they are translocation carriers.

Families with chromosomal disorders are often relieved to learn that either chromosomal nondisjunction or chromosomal rearrangement is responsible for the problem. They frequently summarize the information by saying, "It's just been an accident, not something wrong with our genes. So I guess it isn't really a genetic thing in our family."

Families seeking counseling for a chromosomal disorder need to learn what genes and chromosomes are and how they differ. Once individuals are clear about genes and chromosomes, the counselor can explain about meiosis (without necessarily using that term) and how misdivisions can occur during this process. If the family is concerned about a translocation, the counselor will show pictures of the translocation and how different types of gametes can be formed. Obviously, diagrams are extremely useful in both these explanations.

Some individuals may need a quick review about what happens at conception (i.e., the egg and sperm join). Parents are frequently relieved to learn that (except for some cases of mosaicism), chromosomal constitution of the fetus is determined at the time of conception, thus dispelling lingering doubts and fears that they have caused their child's problem through an activity or misdeed during pregnancy.

The frequency of chromosomal disorders due to segregational errors during meiosis increases as maternal age increases. Recent studies utilizing quinacrine fluorescent polymorphic variants have shown that the extra chromosome in Down's syndrome was paternal in origin in one-third of the cases (Stene et al. 1977). The parent who has contributed the abnormal germ cell is generally not identifiable. By giving parents information about increased risk with increasing maternal age, and pointing out that there is no proof of which parent contributed the abnormal gamete in their particular case, neither parent need assume full responsibility for that child's disorder, yet both are made aware of increasing risks in future pregnancies.

For all known chromosomal and some Mendelian disorders, amniocentesis can be used for prenatal diagnosis. This means a couple can elect to have an affected fetus aborted. In discussing amniocentesis with prospective parents, the genetic counselor needs to caution them that it cannot detect small chromosomal rearrangements or the presence of deleterious genes (other than the one for which the test is being specifically made).

Couples need to be informed about amniocentesis, but not at the expense of a careful genetic explanation as well. Since amniocentesis is one of the few ways in which genetic counselors can offer certitudes about pregnancies instead of probabilities, it is not surprising that genetic counselors want to get to a discussion of this technique quickly. In some cases the couple has heard about amniocentesis and wants to discuss it first. If the genetic counselor remembers to return to the genetic explanation, an early discussion of amniocentesis can work well. If the couple has not heard of amniocentesis, the counselor may want to point out that there is a test for future pregnancies that he or she would like to discuss after the genetic explanation has been given. The knowledge that there is a test sometimes helps individuals to relax and focus on the genetic explanation.

Dominant Disorders

In counseling for dominant disorders, the genetic counselor confronts different situations, depending on whether a parent or prospective parent carries the dominant gene, or whether the gene is a new mutation in a child. A parent or prospective parent with a dominant gene often feels a conflict between the desire to have a child, and the need to be reassured that the child will be healthy. Since the recurrence risk is 50 percent if a parent has the dominant gene, the conflict can be very strong. For example, one man with Charcot-Marie-Tooth disease was unsure he wanted to have a child: "One side is the birth defect thing. Not so much over guilt, but how sensitive is it of me to have a child that may end up that way? I have no need to prove myself in that manner." His wife, who wanted a child very much, also felt the conflict, but in a different way:

> I feel that if we had a child that was affected, it would put my husband through a lot of feelings of responsibility and guilt. I don't feel that I could do that to him unless he was *really* wanting a child and willing to take the risk as much as I am.

Sometimes the spouse of a person with a dominant gene is unwilling to take the risk of having a child with it. In these cases, unaffected spouses face a dilemma. If they don't speak up, their spouse will assume they are willing to take the 50 percent risk; if they do speak up, their affected spouse may feel rejected. The following exchange occurred between a man with Alport's syndrome and his wife:

JIM: I'm saying I should be considered worthy given the state of condition I have, so the child that has the same thing should also be considered worthy. So you reject him, you reject me.

ANN: I think that I often don't come on strong because I am afraid that you are going to take it as a rejection of you.

JIM: True.

In some cases, genetic counseling for dominant genetic disorders is made more difficult by incomplete penetrance (i.e., the trait commonly associated with that disorder is absent in both parents, so one cannot be sure the gene is present) or incomplete expressivity (i.e., the trait varies in severity of expression, as in high-frequency or complete hearing loss in Wardenburg's syndrome). When penetrance and expressivity are incomplete, prospective parents may have no first-hand experience with the disease, making their decision a more difficult one. Also, they might feel comfortable taking a 50 percent chance of having a child with high-frequency hearing loss, but not of having a deaf child.

The explanation of dominant inheritance is straightforward, with capital letters customarily used to depict the dominant or "stronger" gene "that causes problems." If counselees have little biologic background, it is not necessary to introduce the term "chromosome." Instead, the counselor can say, "Individuals get one copy of each gene, or genetic information, from each parent, so each person has two copies of each gene. Since Richard has Charcot-Marie-Tooth disease, we know he has C (for the Charcot-Marie-Tooth Disease) and c for his other gene." The types of offspring expected can then be explained using cc for his wife's genes.

The person with the dominant disorder often looks pleased and relieved to learn that everyone carries a genetic load of from three to five genes, any one of which, if combined with a gene like itself, would cause either abnormality or death. As one woman with a dominant disorder said, "I'm just more up front about my genes, right?"

When a child has a new dominant mutation, parents may have difficulty believing that their genes are not responsible for the child's problems. A careful explanation of mutations and mutation rate will suffice, *if* parents have first grasped such concepts as gene and germ cell. To explain the recurrence risk to the child's future children, the genetic counselor will use c and C to represent their child's genes for the trait and cc for the probable spouse's genes. (Unless individuals are very knowledgeable about genetics, the term "alleles" need not be introduced.)

Recessive Disorders

Although carrier tests for such diseases as Tay-Sachs and sickle cell disease can now give some parents advance warning that they are at an increased risk of having an affected child, most parents are not aware that they are carriers until an affected child is born. Parents who were not aware of their carrier status usually seek genetic counseling shortly after the birth of an affected child, and are likely to be still in shock. In some cases, both spouses shoulder the responsibility equally. In others, dissension even involves the grandparents: "My father particularly was concerned about which side of the family the Tay-Sachs gene came from and was *sure* that it was not his side. And he *still* will maintain that it must be my mother." Explanations about transmission of a recessive gene are made in much the same way as for a dominant gene. If individuals have little knowledge of biology, the genetic counselor can say that each person has two copies of each gene: one from his or her mother, and one from his or her father. Recessive genes can be described as "weaker" or "not as strong as" normal genes. In diagrams or other visual aids, lower case letters are used to denote the recessive gene and capital letters, the normal. Whenever possible, the genetic counselor should avoid the use of the term *normal* when contrasting it to the dominant or recessive allele. Instead, phrases such as "the usual form," "the type of gene commonly found," "found in most people" are more comfortable for the person with the problem to hear. A description of the genetic load carried by everyone is useful in such cases and can help keep carriers of recessive genes from feeling "rare" or "singled out." If the individuals have no children or have a very young affected child, some time may have to be spent acquainting them with the disease and its ramifications before they can make an informed decision concerning reproduction. Some counselors use films of affected children; others know families with affected children of varying ages who are happy to talk to prospective parents.

X-linked Disorders   When a disease is X-linked (e.g., hemophilia, Duchenne's muscular dystrophy), it soon becomes obvious to families that the disorder is passed from mother to son. It is the mother or prospective mother who is tested for carrier status and whose family history is most carefully noted.

Although the counselor may say that no one is to blame and that being a carrier is not within a person's control, it is not surprising that women often feel they are "the only one responsible." In addition to some feelings of guilt, carrier women have often had prior experiences with the disease through affected brothers and uncles, giving them a different perspective of the disease than that of their husbands. Although some carrier women have realized for some time that they could be carriers, it can still be a shock to get the definitive test results, as one carrier for hemophilia pointed out: "I always felt I was a carrier. But it still came as a startling thing to hear the test results, you know." Therefore, informing women that they are carriers needs to be done in a gentle, slow, and compassionate manner. Many carriers of X-linked disorders are relieved to learn that all human beings (including their husbands), carry deleterious genes. One woman said, "When can I bring in my husband? He'll believe it if you tell him."

In addition to genes and chromosomes, a basic explanation of X-linked disorders must include a discussion about how the sex of a child is determined. For example, the genetic counselor might say:

As you know, the sex of a child is determined at the time of conception by genetic material contributed from both the egg (from the mother) and the sperm (from the father). The mother's cells that make the eggs have two sex determining chromosomes called XX. When eggs are made, the cells divide so that each egg receives one of the mother's X' s—only one.

The sperm is derived from the father's cells that contain genetic material called X and Y. He has an X that is like a women's X, but also a Y—the Y is responsible for him being a man. In making sperm, the father's cells divide so that each sperm gets *either* an X *or* a Y. It cannot get both.

If an X from the mother's egg joins with an X from the father's sperm, there will be a girl baby. If an X from the mother joins with a Y from the father, there will be a boy baby.

The counselor can then continue to talk about the two kinds of boy babies (affected and normal) and girl babies (carrier and normal), making use of diagrams in which one of the mother's X's is marked.

The above description was given in its simplest terms. Depending on the background of the individuals counseled, and the questions they ask, more detail can be added. In general, it is better to make a simple explanation and to add details later.

Couples in which the woman is a carrier for an X-linked disorder can avoid having an affected male child by aborting all males. This is a difficult decision for many people, since there is a 50 percent chance that the male child will not be affected. Also, some couples are reluctant to have only female children. One husband of an X-linked carrier said: "Well, you know, a man always just traditionally was more interested in having a male—more concerned about having male children."

Polygenic Disorders   Increasingly, the relatives of individuals with polygenic disorders such as cleft lip or palate, diabetes, or early atherosclerosis are concerned about the risk of these diseases to themselves and their children. Genetic counseling can be more difficult for polygenic than for Mendelian or chromosomal disorders. Although the recurrence risk to first degree relatives is generally low (3–5 percent for birth defects and 5–15 percent for diabetes, according to Motulsky, 1975), this probability of recurrence is based on empiric risk figures. For many diseases the empiric risks are either not available or are incomplete, especially when several first degree relatives are affected. Also, environmental factors play a large role in the expression of these diseases. Explanations about the inheritance of polygenic diseases need to start with a clear description of the genes. The description need not be technical—e.g., "the substances that determine how our bodies will develop and grow." Counselees need to know that a fetus receives half its genes from one parent and half from the other, and that different children in the same family receive a different set of genes from each parent. It then becomes possible for people to understand that a certain total number of genes in a fetus (e.g., seven) can result in the presence of a cleft lip, and that some of these genes have come from each parent (e.g., three from one and four from the other, or two from one and five from the other).

When empiric risk figures are available, they should, of course, be used in genetic counseling, but not at the expense of the genetic explanation, or of discussion with the concerned individuals. One woman who sought genetic counseling for juvenile diabetes said of her diagnostic visit: "It just seemed so kind of dry. The genetic counselor just pulled out this paper and there it was. Everything was on one piece of paper that he just carries around." This woman was reacting more to the abrupt manner in which she was given the information than to the genetic counselor having the information written down. Generally, people are pleased that a genetic counselor will take the time to research information or write down specific facts and figures for them to take home.

Diagnosis Uncertain Sometimes a diagnosis cannot be made. Either the available medical records are incomplete (e.g., baby died, hospital records burned) or there is at present no possible diagnosis, despite ample medical records (e.g., some types of mental retardation). If there is an absent or inconclusive family history for the problem, it is sometimes not possible to determine whether the birth defect in question is "an accident in development" due to nongenetic causes (recurrence probably less than 0.05 percent), a new mutation (recurrence risk almost 0), a polygenic disorder (about five percent recurrence risk), recessive genes (25 percent recurrence risk), or an X-linked gene (50 percent risk for male offspring, 25 percent for all offspring).

Understandably, parents want more certain information on which they can base their future reproductive and child raising decisions. Some couples are overwhelmed by the uncertainty and may become angry, depressed, or withdraw from counseling altogether if the genetic counselor has not built a firm basis of trust in earlier visits.

When there is no diagnosis, there is often no prognosis either. Since the child has an unrecognizable syndrome, it may not be possible to accurately predict what he or she can or cannot do in the next few years. A father of a mentally retarded child with an uncertain diagnosis reflected:

> As long as she isn't diagnosed, we don't know what can be done for her. Now my cousin has a Down's syndrome kid and we know what the prognosis is. I mean, you can teach him something. But the limitations are pretty well known. We don't know the limitations on Alice.

When it is not possible to give parents a prognosis, they need time to express their disappointment that there is no more to be learned, and to test whether they have clearly understood that there is at present no more information available. The mother of a mentally retarded child said: "I want somebody to give me results. Not just take him there and then, 'Well, we can't help you.' I'm sick of that and I want to know why or what I can do!" Unless parents are allowed to express their frustration in this manner, to ask for information in several ways, and to finally accept that the genetic counselor has given them all of the currently available information, they may assume that the genetic counselor doesn't care enough to really find out what the problem is, and may look elsewhere for help.

Parents of a child with an uncertain diagnosis need to be carefully shown that the genetic counselor is in a position to know about new syndromes (or be referred to a specialist who is), and that the counselor is aware of the latest research in the field. In addition, the genetic counselor can point out that new advances in genetics and medicine occur almost daily, and can offer to put the family's name in a file to be notified when a pertinent development occurs.

Such comments show that the genetic counselor is interested in the family, and provide some hope for the future. Without hope for even modest gains in the future, many people have difficulty accepting the present. More immediately, the family should be made aware of social agencies, special schools, physical therapy programs, etc., appropriate for their problem.

Perhaps most importantly, the genetic counselor should

remember to include the parents in the diagnostic process. First, parents may have observations which may facilitate the diagnosis. Second, it is an enormous boost to the parents' morale to learn that they can help. The father of a child with delayed developmental milestones said:

> I think that both of us can help the doctors quite a bit. That's what happened last time. They asked a lot of questions about what *we* observed from him. And I think watching his development the way we have, we could help quite a bit and they might even be able to tell us something more.

Probability and Statistics
Even when a diagnosis can be made, when the family history unequivocally shows that there is a genetic disease present, when the genetic counselor can tell individuals the mode of inheritance, much genetic counseling information is given in probabilistic fashion. That is, if both parents are carriers for the same recessive gene, there is a 25 percent chance with each conception that the child will be affected. There is no certain knowledge about the outcome of any particular pregnancy, however.

In addition to being uncertain, statistics are difficult for people in other ways. Some people consider 25 percent high and others low, depending on how they evaluate the seriousness of the disease. Not only do different people rank diseases differently (including genetic counselors, see Sorenson, 1973), but the same people can differ in their appraisal of a disease over a period of time:

> For me, I think a risk figure would vary with what place my life was in at the time. If we were in the middle of this upheaval and it was fifty percent, I don't think that would be good enough for me. Even eighty percent wouldn't be good enough for me at that time. But I could be in the middle of a beautiful period and 10 percent would feel OK.

An understanding of the meaning of a probability in one's own life is not dependent on either education or intelligence. Even individuals whom one would expect to be knowledgeable about numbers can become quite confused when faced with making decisions about risk in their own lives. For example, a mathematician who was concerned about the possible deleterious effects of his consanguinous marriage said: "I know that 10 percent is in actuality only one percent more than nine percent, and yet nine *sounds* like a very much lower number compared to 10." Some people, like one prospective parent, want children so strongly that they will not decide before genetic counseling what would constitute a high risk for them:

> I don't know. I can't decide. I guess I'd rather wait and find out what you say and then decide. I'd hate to say 30 percent chance and above is it—we won't have children. Because I don't know. That just seems so final. Maybe I'm just not ready to accept the fact that there's a chance that we wouldn't want to have children.

Still others will say, "I don't follow percentages too closely."

There is no one way to make probability and statistics meaningful. However, the genetic counselor's chances of doing so are increased if he or she learns the individuals' main concerns about the genetic disease and creates an environment in which individuals feel comfortable about asking for clarification.

To teach probability, the chance of getting heads or tails when flipping a coin is often used. Some couples seem to understand probability in relation to future pregnancies when a biologic example is used, e.g., the chance that a child's sex will be male (50 percent probability) or female (50 percent). The counselor can then point out that although the chance of having a boy is fifty percent for each pregnancy, we all know families in which there are two girls or four girls, and only one boy. Whatever method is used to make probability relevant, care should be taken to ascertain whether individuals understand that the events of one pregnancy have no bearing on another. That is, the birth of an affected or unaffected child does not mean that the couple's chances of having a normal or affected child in the next pregnancy are any different from the probability originally given. Many people seem to think that having one genetic problem predisposes them to having another, even of a completely different type.

People can repeat the risk figures the genetic counselor has given them without understanding the implication and relevance of these figures in their own lives. Therefore, the genetic counselor may need several follow-up visits with a family to check whether they have grasped the implications of the risk figures given.

5 Follow-up Visits

I am now deeply convinced, and more and more of my colleagues who work with parents seem to agree, that it takes a series of sessions, spread out over several months, before most parents come even somewhat to grips with the nature and, particularly, the implications of a diagnosis.

Time and again one finds that not even parents with professional and mental health backgrounds, nor those who profess a verbal understanding during the first feedback session, have even made a good start in working through their conflicts. For this reason, spaced and repeated feedback counseling should be viewed not as a luxury but as an integral part of the function of a diagnostic service. Such counseling should be offered even if it necessitates case load reduction since, in the long run, it will probably conserve professional manpower. It is penny-wise and pound-foolish to invest substantial and valuable resources into the diagnostic process only to begrudge a few additional hours of counseling. If the parents are not adequately counseled, they may not only go shopping, but perhaps even worse, their defenses may harden and may render them inaccessible to help. In the end this may cost ten, a hundred and even a thousandfold what a few hours of counseling would have cost.

W. Wolfensberger, 1965

Increasingly, genetic counselors are beginning to note the necessity of follow-up visits. However, due to a shortage of staff, follow-up visits are not always offered as a routine part of genetic counseling services. Instead, they are made available "for those who really need them," or "if it seems necessary." When individuals seeking genetic counseling realize that follow-up visits are not routine, they frequently feel awkward about availing themselves of such visits. They may feel that follow-up visits are a confirmation of their inability to deal with the situation or that they have been singled out for special treatment. Some people are concerned about taking up too much of the genetic counselor's time or even of depriving others whom they feel may have greater needs. For many people, to ask for additional help means they are failures and they suffer a loss of self-esteem. For these and other reasons, follow-up visits, to be successful, need to be an integral part of the genetic counseling service.

Areas Covered in Follow-up Visits

The genetic counselor will have evolved a tentative agenda for the first follow-up based on issues raised in previous visits.* Although the specifics of each one vary, based on the nature of each case and the individuals involved, the following areas will generally be covered in follow-up visits:

What Has Been Happening to and Within the Family Since the Last Genetic Counseling Session

The counselor will want to make his or her own note about how each family member looks compared to the last visit. Are they more relaxed or more tense? Do they have fewer or more questions than the counselor would expect? Are they more or less happy than expected, given the nature of the information they have received?

Sometimes the genetic counselor will comment on the family's unexpected reactions to the information they have received. This may serve to reveal whether the individuals have correctly understood the information given or it may serve to open a dialogue between the parents. For example, the following exchange occurred during a first follow-up visit with parents of a retarded child who had previously expressed a desire to have more children:

HOWARD: Well, they said that it was nothing genetic. I mean like as far as us having babies, they said go ahead. You know, the chance of something like this happening again would be very slight if any at all.

MARY: I don't want any more kids anyway. Not even one. I did before, but I don't want any more.

KELLY: I'm surprised. How did you arrive at that?

*A follow-up interview guide is given in Appendix A.

The wife then went on to explain her hesitations about having another child. Her explanation served to assure the genetic counselor that her decision, though surprising, was indeed based on comprehension of the diagnostic information.

What Each Person Has Learned from the Diagnostic Visit

Frequently, people do not fully understand what they were told during the diagnostic visit. The fault may be neither theirs nor the genetic counselor's, but can be due to anxiety on the part of individuals seeking genetic counseling. Also, the technical nature of much genetic counseling information can preclude immediate understanding even for geneticists. The genetic counselor will therefore want to check up on what information individuals actually heard and understood. Sometimes individuals want to know why the genetic counselor asks about what they were previously told in as much as the counselor was present during the diagnostic visit or has access to the records. For example:

KELLY: Well, tell me what happened. What went on?

DICK: Well, you must know as much as I do. You were in that, that conference. I don't know any more than that. I haven't heard a word since.

KELLY: That's right. I was there. And there was so much going on, so much said, that I wanted to see what was important to you out of all that was going on.

In this way, the genetic counselor makes it plain that the individual is not expected to remember everything and that not all of the information is of equal importance. What people do remember is emphasized by the genetic counselor and used to expand their understanding. As people relate what they have understood, the genetic counselor will want to ask how they first felt on hearing the information, how they now feel about the information, and perhaps what brought about the change in feeling or perception.

Sometimes then, people will admit that they did not understand or listen to much of the information. One woman whose child had been stillborn said: "But to tell you the truth, once I heard that it would probably never happen again, the statistics didn't stick. That's just what I wanted to hear and that was it." Usually, it is advisable at this point to recapitulate the salient facts (including the statistics) with the family, since they will want them at a future time. As time passes, some people may begin to worry that they may not have heard all of the relevant information during the counseling session or that the genetic counselor may not have investigated every aspect of their case. Follow-up letters, as mentioned in Chapter 2, serve a useful function in these instances, in that they remind individuals of the areas covered and information discussed.

What Are the Implications and Ramifications of the Information They Have Received

The genetic counselor will want to learn what the information has meant to individuals. That is, how will they use the information? As discussed in Chapter 9, Questions Genetic Counselors Ask, people frequently change their minds about how they will use genetic counseling information. The first follow-up visit is a good time to learn and record what their reactions were to the information received during the diagnostic visit and to help them explore the implications of their current understanding and decisions. The genetic counselor, who has experience with the effects of genetic disease, can frequently point out issues and areas that counselees have not considered.

What Have Been the Responses of Friends and Relatives

Frequently, friends and relatives ask questions about the prognosis and inheritance of the disease that had not occurred to the individuals seeking counseling. Sometimes friends and relatives have their own theories about the disease that conflict with what individuals were told during genetic counseling. In such cases, the genetic counselor needs to restate the genetic information so it is credible, without disparaging either friends or relatives.

Individuals will occasionally report that they have not told friends and relatives about the disease or about the genetic implications of the disease. An exploration of why parents have not told others can give both genetic counselor and counseled individuals valuable information. If the reticence stems from embarrassment about the disease, as is often the case, the genetic counselor can explore the basis of the embarrassment. Sometimes it becomes evident that the reason individuals have not told friends and relatives about the genetic disease was because they do not fully understand the information. To reach such an understanding may take several visits. One man had had three follow-up visits in which the genetic, medical, and social aspects of his daughter's illness had been discussed. During the fourth visit he suddenly turned and said:

> Thank you, thank you for telling me why our daughter died. I have wondered and not understood it. When my friends asked, I was so embarrassed because I couldn't tell them why. I felt I was to blame. Now that you have told me, I can tell them.

The timing and number of follow-up visits needed are variable and depend on the counselor's perception of need as well as the individuals who seek genetic counseling. Two follow-up visits are sufficient in some cases, while four may be too few in others. Sometimes individuals will have a crisis in their family lives, or become concerned about a new aspect of the disease, and will feel an urgent need to talk to the genetic counselor again. This need may be felt six months or as long as a year and a half after the last follow-up visit. Usually the initial follow up is held one to three weeks after the diagnostic visit. This interval gives people time to think about the information they have received and to get feedback from friends and relatives. Frequently people report that the sound and meaning of the information changes between the genetic counseling session and the retelling in their own home.

The Main Purposes of Follow-up Visits

To Check on Individuals' Understanding of the Information They Have Received

Individuals' anxieties and the technical nature of much genetic counseling information often necessitate several visits to achieve understanding.

To Help Individuals Integrate the Information into Their Lives

To achieve this integration, which means fitting the general information into the specifics of their lives, individuals often need to talk about the information and try out the various alternatives. For example, one woman who learned she was a carrier for Tay-Sachs disease said of her first follow-up:

> It was good to talk about it. There hasn't been anybody who's said to me, "What are your thoughts about it?" It's a good thing to have said—and to be able to talk about. And there were questions that you asked that I had to think about.

Another person said: "It's nice to be able to sit here now having gone through it all and tell you our troubles and our fears and the good things about it." Of course, while telling the genetic counselor, people are frequently becoming clearer about how the material sounds to them. Since the genetic counselor has had previous experience with similar cases, he or she can frequently help people in this integration process.

The genetic counselor also helps by being able to inform individuals of various alternatives that are possible in a given situation. It is not infrequent for individuals to forget about one alternative because they were concentrating on another at the time alternatives were first introduced. Also, alternatives that seemed unacceptable at first can become more tolerable as people become accustomed to them. More than this, genetic counselors also help focus discussions so that the issues and alternatives can be clearly considered. During a follow-up, one woman said:

> I would like a little more direction than somebody just saying, "Well, there's a 3 percent chance that you'll have some kind of genetic difficulty." I would like some *direction*. Is that really a large chance? And what does that mean in reality?

Comments such as this indicate that individuals would like to explore the ramifications of the information they have heard.

In addition to clarifying issues and information, the genetic counselor furthers the integration process by helping individuals to maintain open communication. This may involve neutralizing vindictive comments by relatives who seek to blame one member of a couple, or encouraging individuals to tell each other about their feelings about the disease. Freeman (1971) notes that it is natural for one member of a couple to be reticent about raising issues that might cause the other pain or embarrassment. However, if these issues are not discussed, misunderstandings can arise or people can lose touch with each other. In such circumstances, satisfactory integration and application of the information may become impossible. Therefore, during follow-ups, a major aim of the genetic counselor is to maintain open communication.

To Make Appropriate Referrals

For specifics about how to refer people to a mental health professional, see Chapter 9. The counselor may also think it advisable to refer people to physical therapists, social service agencies of various sorts, or public health nurses, etc. Referral can be a most important service, since individuals who come for genetic counseling frequently do not know what services might be available. (e.g., special schools or classes, homemaker services). Also, knowledge about what kinds of social services are and are not available can shape individuals' decisions.

The transcript of a follow-up visit that follows illustrates a number of issues that frequently arise in these sessions. A reading of this transcript convincingly demonstrates the essential role of follow-up visits. If it takes a couple who received good news during the diagnostic visit a full follow-up visit to assimilate the information, how much more necessary are such visits when the information involves more uncertainty or is unwelcome! Therefore, it is essential that genetic counseling services schedule follow-up visits and not assume that information can generally be assimilated during the diagnostic visit, even if the information seems simple or straightforward.

The transcript that follows has been edited to remove repetitions and to clarify statements. However, no substantive changes have been made. A husband (Henry) and wife (Jane) met with the author (Kelly). This couple had had their intake visit with the author and their diagnostic visit with a physician (Dr. Evans) who diagnosed the wife as having oculocutaneous albinism. The author's comments and analysis of the process of the session have been interpolated in italics in appropriate places.

Transcript of a Follow-up Visit

KELLY: (To Henry) How's it been since I saw you? I talked to Jane on the phone.

[*The genetic counselor starts with a general question.*]

HENRY: Well, I was very happy with our meeting with Dr. Evans, and we've talked about it a lot since then. Well, especially right after. I think one of the reasons I was pleased with it is because I hadn't seen all the doctors, known all the things she had found out and Jane didn't repeat to me everything that she's learned since she was a kid.

[*This is a good reason to request that spouses be present for all parts of a genetic counseling session.*]

HENRY: (continuing) But it was nice for me to understand what Jane's problem was. See, one of the things I thought before we came to the clinic was that it would be difficult to determine whether or not her problem was in fact a genetic problem or to what extent it was genetic and what extent it was due to other factors which weren't clearly heredity. And apparently the doctor was convinced that her eye problems were related to what he called generalized albinism. I think that was the word he gave it. So it was nice for me to understand, for example, that her problems came from a genetic thing and not from say, using her eyes too much at work or something like that.

[*Here Henry is pointing out that they had not realized that Jane's eye problems were related to her fair skin.*]

KELLY: Well then you could feel you didn't have to worry about it right now because she is the way she is. Is that what you're saying?

HENRY: Yes. Well, see this way I don't feel that she's going to be getting worse because of some gradually deteriorating situation. In other words, if you understand what the disorder is, you can maybe have a better idea of what the prognosis will be. I realize this isn't so much related to having a child, but it was one of the things that I was happy to get out of talking with the doctor.

[*To many people seeking genetic counseling, the prognosis is of primary importance since it enables them to better understand what to expect from the disease in the future.*]

KELLY: Yes. I can see that. Jane, did you know that Henry used to worry about you? That he thought that your eyes might get worse?

[*Here the genetic counselor is checking to see if Jane was aware of her husband's concern. It is also a way to bring Jane into the conversation.*]

JANE: Well sure! Because even I was never that certain about what was going on. You know, when we came in we thought that they were two separate problems: being fair and not being able to see too well. What I found out was that they were inextricably connected and that you can't talk about one without the other. *I* never even understood it. And the reason Henry didn't understand it was because I didn't. And I never really understood quite as well as I do now. It was sort of a coming together of all sorts of facts. I think what really astounded me was how Dr. Evans didn't have any reservations or any doubts about what was wrong.

[*The genetic counselor not only must be able to make the diagnosis, he or she must be able to convince individuals that it is correct.*]

JANE: (continuing) And I told him so. Because most other doctors I've seen would say, "I'm not an expert in genetics," or, "I don't know everything about your family." They would always leave a little leeway so they wouldn't say 100 percent that they were sure about what it was or about what would happen in terms of children. Even in that he was completely certain and I was amazed by it.

KELLY: What did he say when you told him you were amazed?

[This can be a way to determine if the individual has told the doctor her feelings about the diagnosis. In cases where she has not, it is clearly important to go over those aspects that are still amazing, surprising, etc.]

JANE: (pause) I thought maybe my telling him that I thought it was unusual or saying, "Come on, come on. It couldn't be all that rosy," would make him say, "Well, I don't want to misdeceive you. It's really a 5 percent risk I'm talking about." Or something. But he wouldn't. In fact, I kept going over that and saying, "How sure are you of your numbers?" He seemed to be unshakable about it, which was kind of a shock.

What we've talked about at home is trying to go over that again and figuring out what the odds are exactly.

[The genetic counselor who conducted the diagnostic visit may have felt that the couple had absorbed as much information as they could at that time and therefore did not dwell on the figures. Or, Jane may not have been able to concentrate on the quantitative aspects then. Note that Jane paused before replying. Such pauses can be quite useful in allowing individuals to collect their thoughts.]

JANE: (continuing) Even though in the interview he made it very personal and very human and didn't go into numbers first of all, but rather said, "If your question is, do you run the risk of having an albino child, don't worry about it; go ahead and have children." And he made it very qualitative. And that registered and that made an impact. I think when we went home, we thought about that and we also thought about the quantitative part. And I kept thinking, "Well, exactly what are the odds?"

[Note that Jane speaks of her diagnostic visit as an interview, not as a medical visit. Many who seek genetic counseling do not consider themselves to be patients.]

HENRY: Well, if I could interrupt. He did make quantitative statements. I think what Jane means is that the general mood of the discussion was one of encouragement.

[As the session unfolds, it becomes apparent that the genetic counselor had provided the quantitative aspects. Jane had not been able to focus on them at that time. Before concluding that

counselees have not heard information, it is wise to let the session continue a bit.]

HENRY: (continuing) But I wouldn't want to give the impression that he didn't try to be specific . . .

JANE: He did. He did. He did a really good job.

KELLY: Well, what did you get out of it specifically?

[*The genetic counselor wants to learn more about what each of them heard and now remembers—in specific terms.*]

JANE: Um . . . (pause)

[*The genetic counselor clarifies her question, having decided that the pause had continued long enough.*]

KELLY: I guess what I'd like to hear about is what happened. What diagnosis did he give you? What numbers did he give you? What did you come away with?

HENRY: Have you consulted with him about it or . . . ?

KELLY: Yes.

HENRY: Oh, so you just want to hear from our side?

JANE: What we got out of it?

[*The genetic counselor explains why it is important to hear about the information from Jane and Henry, without making it sound like a quiz.*]

KELLY: What he told you is not necessarily what you got out of it. I mean what you get out of it, Henry, is not necessarily what Jane gets out of it.

[*Here the genetic counselor points out that Henry and Jane may differ in their understanding and reaction to the information they received during the diagnostic visit.*]

HENRY: Yeah. Yeah.

KELLY: So that's really more what I'm interested in.

JANE: I'd like to hope that the content of all three of our (laughs) recollections are close.

[*Jane might be worried that she has forgotten some of the information. Note that Jane's comment can be interpreted more sternly without the laugh.*]

JANE: (continuing) I got out of it that I shouldn't worry about it. That the incidence in the population is extremely low and the probability that Henry would have a recessive gene that would produce an albino baby is *really* low. And I shouldn't even be concerned about worrying about it. *However*, I've been used to worrying about it for so long, I'm not sure it's that easy to just stop it and erase it.

[*Jane illustrates an important issue here. If an individual has held an idea or concern, it can be difficult to give up that concern on an emotional level, regardless of the rational explanation provided.*]

JANE: (continuing) But that's what he said and, of course, I was really happy to hear that.

He looked at me, shined a little light in my eyes and asked me questions about my past and my present. I think most of the time he did spend explaining to us exactly what it was and then answering the question which was what risk do we have. He said that it was a treat for him because it's not too often he gets to tell people such good news. And, as I said earlier, he was really unqualified in his answer of, "Yes. Go ahead." It was very nice, the whole time. It almost seemed too good to be true.

KELLY: Well, how does it seem now? You've had a couple of weeks now.

[*The genetic counselor is wondering how much of the information they now believe and what further questions they have.*]

JANE: (pause) Well, naturally some of the details fade away, just because your memory isn't that perfect. I guess my last statement reflects how I really feel. It's good news. I probably have more qualms than he has.

HENRY: Than me or the doctor?

[*When the tempo of genetic counseling sessions is unhurried, the couple or family has an opportunity to interact.*]

JANE: Than the doctor had. Probably than you too, which is why I kept making Henry go over the numbers. I think in my *soul*, my *heart*, I believe him. Because I can tell from my dreaming or from my worries just as I'm starting to wake up. But my rationality gets in the way and I keep looking for the loophole that he forgot or the equation that doesn't add up. So I made Henry get a piece of paper out and we tried to work it out again to prove it.

I had a telephone call from my mother. And I told her about the genetic counseling. This was about two weeks after it. And her reply was. . . . I was startled. But it was, "Don't be too sure. That's not what I understand the facts to be. Your odds are probably 50–50." And she was. . . .

[*Friends and relatives frequently have ideas about the inheritance of genetic diseases that differ from the information given during genetic counseling.*]

KELLY: Wow!

[*The genetic counselor wants to register her surprise at the high risk figure Jane's mother expressed.*]

JANE: Yes. So. Okay. I didn't want to get into it. In fact, when I was talking to her, I was trying it on different levels. I was trying it qualitatively. I was trying it quantitatively. And everything she said was factually correct as far as inheritance of dominant and recessive, etc. So I sat down and I wrote her a long letter and I tried to explain it to her. In fact, I figured it out—our odds, given that Henry is typical of somebody in the population who doesn't necessarily have this gene. Dr. Evans told us that the odds were one in 300 that someone would have the gene. I tried to show her with little equations how our odds were at least three times greater of having a normal baby than their odds were after they had me and found out that they each had a recessive. And I don't think she's used to thinking about it that way. Of course, I'm not either 'cause I had to make Henry sit down and help me figure it all out again. I think now I've finally got it straight, but for a while it was easy for me to forget the logic of how it all worked and panic and think, "Oh my God! Wait a minute. You might be that person."

[*Jane has periods of doubt.*]

JANE: (continuing) And he said, "Well, wait a minute, there are 299 chances that I'm not." And I'd go through it again. I think finally I've got it down as far as the math and I want to understand the math.

[*Note that Jane, like many genetic counseling clients, feels differently when the risk figures are expressed in their reverse form.*]

KELLY: Yes. I can see why. But I wonder, though, if your mother's saying something else. You know: "It happened to me."

[*The genetic counselor feels that going over the math again at this point will be less valuable than confronting emotional reactions to the new information. One way to approach the wife's doubt on an emotional level is by discussing her mother's doubt.*]

JANE: Sure. She seems fearful.
HENRY: A sort of emotional thing.

[*Note that Henry agrees that the mother's reaction is an emotional one.*]

JANE: She gave me a barbed thing like, "Of course, you can do whatever you want. It's your life", which is a very stinging thing to say. Meaning, "I wouldn't do it. Are you sure?"

HENRY: The ironic thing is that she realized after she had Jane that there was a problem. Apparently she talked to someone, I don't think a geneticist, and was even told that it was from a recessive gene. Of course, given that her parents would know that they both have recessives, you don't have to worry about the one in 300 odds anymore; it's one out of four then for them. Even so, she went on ahead and had more children. And when Jane mentioned that one out of four, her mother said, "Yeah, they said one out of four." And apparently believes that Jane's little sister also has the same problem. Now I don't know whether that's true or not.

JANE: She said in case you were wondering, my little sister is undisputably diagnosed the way Dr. Evans would diagnose somebody. That's why it was brought up again now. Just in case you think you're off the hook, your little sister has it too and that makes it worse. Of course, my sister's genes or my genes don't change Henry's genes.

KELLY: It sounds like your mother's having a hard time right now.

[*The genetic counselor is careful not to dismiss the mother's concerns.*]

JANE: Well, of course, I felt real badly because when I hung up, nothing was resolved. So I sat down and wrote her this letter and it will be interesting to see what she says. She's not a stupid woman and she has taken a lot of courses in biology and genetics and I think pictures in her mind a little square where you put rr on one side and Rr on the vertical side and if you do that you get a 50% chance of having an albino baby. . . .

HENRY: What she's missing is the course in statistics that she needs to round out her knowledge.

KELLY: She's assuming then that Henry also has the recessive?

[*The genetic counselor turns the conversation back to the issue of whether Henry is a carrier of the albino gene.*]

JANE: Well, she's saying, "Why would you dare assume otherwise?" The risk is so scary.

[*Jane is spelling out her own concern here.*]

HENRY: See, the assumption is: If I have the risk, meaning her. "If daddy and I have the recessive, we're normal people, we're dark, he must have it too."

JANE: In fact, she says she's afraid for my other married sister. And my sister's husband I'm sure has a one in 300 chance which I don't think my mother appreciates. But I think it's probably the case. And my sister would probably be like my parents. In other words, she isn't affected, so she's probably, definitely a dominant in the one gene and the other gene is either a dominant or a recessive, so her odds are a lot better than Henry's and mine.

[Jane, despite her doubts and protestations of not really understanding the numbers, demonstrates a firm grasp of the genetics.]

JANE: And I can see why it worries them to think of the fact that there could be—there is a possibility that Henry is indeed the—and that is an emotional thing.

[It would be interesting to have Jane complete the last sentence. She probably did not want to call her husband a carrier.]

KELLY: Did Dr. Evans talk to you at all about the fact that there are different kinds of people who are albinos, that there are people who are called tyrosinase positive and some are tyrosinase negative?

[The genetic counselor wants to be sure specific points were understood.]

HENRY: Yes, he mentioned it.
JANE: Yes, but you know, I'm not quite sure what that says. What I thought that meant was that if somebody has no pigment at all, they don't have the enzymes so they're negative. And somebody like me who has a little bit of melanin, has the enzymes so I'm positive. But frankly it looks like he could just look at each of us and say the same thing.
KELLY: Well, what I'm saying is that some people have more problems with lack of pigment than others, more than you do.

[Here the genetic counselor is trying to point out that although Jane is an albino, she will not have some of the difficulties tyrosinase negative albinos have, nor would her children.]

KELLY: (continuing) There are people who don't have pigment in their eyes. It seems that the gene that's in your family and what we're talking about is the other kind. In other words, your eyes are colored. I remembered last time you were talking about albinos and pink eyes.

[Jane had talked about albinos and pink eyes during the intake visit.]

JANE: It's a whole different gene?

KELLY: Yes.

JANE: Oh. I didn't know that.

KELLY: Well, the scientists didn't either until. . . .

JANE: Well, that's neat.

> [*Jane seems relieved. However, the genetic counselor wants to provide proof that the genes are different.*]

KELLY: There were two black people in the South and they were both albinos. They were told, "If you marry, you'll have only albino kids." They did marry, but none of their kids were albino. So they said to the husband, "You couldn't possibly be the father of these kids or they'd be albino." The husband didn't believe it and went from doctor to doctor. They finally discovered that there are two different kinds of recessive albinos and that he was the father of these kids. There were two completely different genes for albinism.

JANE: How could that be?

> [*Jane now wants more information.*]

KELLY: They're on two different places on the chromosomes. They have nothing to do with each other but they produce people that look somewhat alike. So what I'm saying is. . . .

JANE: Oh. Okay. I didn't understand that.

KELLY: Should Henry turn out to be a carrier—which is one in 300—it's pretty low. But if he is a carrier, you might have a child like you. You're not going to have someone with pink eyes and such a little bit of pigment that they can't go outside.

> [*In an earlier visit, Jane had expressed a horror of having a child with pink eyes who couldn't go outside.*]

JANE: Oh, I see.

KELLY: I'm catching that that's what you're worried about. It's a different gene.

JANE: Okay. I'm glad you told me that.

HENRY: Just pursuing that example you gave. Both the black people who were albino, did they have two recessives of this other extreme gene so when they had children they must have. . . . What could they pass on except for recessive? They didn't have any dominant to pass on.

> [*Henry wants technical details, indicating that he has understood most, if not all, of the genetics explained to date.*]

KELLY: Let me show you.

[Here the genetic counselor draws a diagram in which the wife is AAbb and the husband aaBB.]

KELLY: (continuing) So okay, we'll call the negative one *a* and the positive one *b*. And anytime you get a child that's *aa,* that child is going to be an albino. And the *aa* children are going to be much more fair than Jane. No pigment in their eyes. Okay?

JANE AND HENRY: Yes.

KELLY: And the *bb* is going to be like Jane. Two different genes. So we have the lady who was like this (*AAbb*); he was like this (*aaBB*). That's the lady. She was okay for this gene *A* and let's say this *A* was on chromosome six and this *b* was on chromosome seven. Thousands of genes in their 23 pairs of chromosomes. Okay?

HENRY AND JANE: Yes. Okay.

KELLY: Okay. These are completely different genes and you know you have genes for everything from hair color to—everything else. So that's the wife.

HENRY: And she looked like Jane.

KELLY: She looked like Jane. And this is the husband. He was little *a* little *a, aa* and big *B* big *B, BB.* And they got married. The only thing the mother could give was big *A* which she gave. The only thing the father could give was little *a* which he gave.

HENRY: So there was no way they could have an albino.

KELLY: That's right.

[The children were AaBb.]

JANE: Wow!

HENRY: Although the father and the mother must have looked somewhat different because they had different characteristics in the genes.

JANE: These people probably weren't into the subtleties. . . .

HENRY: Right. That's interesting.

JANE: That really is interesting.

HENRY: I was uncertain about this too because it seemed to me, well suppose that Jane had not only the two recessives for what she has but also one recessive for the other problem, and I had one recessive for this other problem, could you have a doubly albino child, something like that who had both problems at once? And also I was wondering that about the sex-linked albinism, the ocular albinism, if you could have that plus one of the others. Do you know about that?

JANE: So there are three kinds. In that case they do not overlap in the parents but, of course, the children each have a recessive of each gene.

KELLY: All of us have from three to five deleterious recessive genes, depending upon whose papers you read. You just happen to know one of the ones that you have.

[Here the genetic counselor wants Jane to realize that everyone has recessive genes, so she is not substantively different from other people. The issue of a doubly recessive child is not confronted directly at this point. When many subjects are raised at once, the genetic counselor can put some aside for later.]

JANE: Well, it's expressed.

KELLY: Yes. All of us have them but they're covered by these other normal ones.

HENRY: Uh hum.

KELLY: For example, I might have one for cystic fibrosis. We're all walking around carrying these genes. But you were asking about overlapping.

[The genetic counselor returns to Henry's question about double albinos.]

KELLY: (continuing) It's so rare, you see, for any of us to have any one of these recessive genes. Eventually we might come upon someone who does have more than one, like the family I told you about, but it would be unlikely.

JANE: There isn't a tendency that if you have one, your probability of having the other two is higher? Or is it so random that it doesn't make any difference?

[Many people wonder if the presence of one genetic problem increases their chances of having others.]

KELLY: That's a good question. I would suspect that it's so random that it doesn't make any difference. We know from animal studies that some genes lie very close to each other, so that if one is present the other is likely to be also. We don't know enough about people, but from what we do know, there's no evidence that your chance of having one albino gene is higher if you have the other.

JANE: Is the incidence of total albinism with the pink eyes the same as mine?

KELLY: It's about the same.

JANE: Because one of the people that my mother kept mentioning to me was a couple who had a completely total baby, without pigment, and when I spoke to her, I thought it was the same gene. You know it's tragic. It's not lethal, but it's still a tragedy. The sex-linked. Is that? Do you think it's possible that it would be a . . . you know.

[Jane is raising some of the issues that have caused her to have doubts.]

KELLY: The sex linked?

[The genetic counselor is unsure about what the question is and so repeats a phrase.]

JANE: Yes. Would it be tied in with my case?

KELLY: The sex-linked we would know from your family. Does your mother have any brothers? I've forgotten. Let's see.

[The genetic counselor looks back at the pedigree chart which was taken during a previous visit.]

KELLY: (continuing) Your mother's brothers would probably show it or your mother's father might show it. It's only these autosomal recessives that can stay hidden for a long time.

JANE: Okay.

KELLY: So if you're going to worry. . . .

JANE: So the sex-linked one is the dominant one. If it's there, it shows?

KELLY: It shows because to make a boy child you have two chromosomes.

[Here the genetic counselor draws a diagram.]

KELLY: (continuing) One's an X and one's a Y. Okay? And to make a girl, there are two X's. And in an X-linked, the X which doesn't have the albino gene covers for the X which has it, in a woman. A man, who gets the X with the albino gene has nothing to cover it with; the Y doesn't cover it.

HENRY: So it's 50–50 for boys.

KELLY: Yes. But girls, if they have the gene, don't usually show it because it's covered. It gets very tricky. There's no greater probability that you have something on your X or any other place than I have or Henry has. Or anybody else in the general population. Nothing higher, and nothing lower, so in that sense, you're just like the rest.

[The genetic counselor tries to stress Jane's normalcy and to show that she is not at increased risk for other genetic diseases.]

JANE: I think you can tell that every once in a while I have second thoughts. Well, what if it happens? Just out of sheer panic. I don't want you to get the impression that I don't trust you, that I don't believe you, 'cause I do. But it's just a question of understanding the nuances of some of the things I didn't really appreciate the first time.

[An excellent summary of some of the uses of a follow-up visit.]

JANE: (continuing) One of the things that I'd like to know, and I realize I'm probably beating the thing to death because as you said. . . .

[The genetic counselor will pick up this phrase later to reassure Jane that her questions are in order.]

JANE: (continuing) We all have from—you said five to 13, you know, some low number of recessive genes. And I hope nothing comes up that we both have recessives, but I realize that I don't want to be too single-minded about it.

[Here Jane is using recessive as a synonym of deleterious. To have corrected her at this point might have impeded the flow of the visit.]

JANE: But in that connection, when you talk about a one in 300 chance. . . . you say that's not very big. Well, if you're going to go gambling, you can appreciate what kinds of odds those are; you probably won't win. But in genetics is that a really big number? In other words, what kinds of other things happen in that kind of range?

[Jane needs help in making the numbers seem real.]

JANE: (continuing) Is there anything greater than one in 300 chance in the general population that I might have to worry about?

KELLY: Sickle cell anemia is much higher. Tay-Sachs disease is much higher. Cystic fibrosis is among certain segments of the population. So the albinism gene isn't considered to be very frequent. No.

HENRY: Is this by any chance correlated more with any segment of the population? Like, let's say, the Jewish population?

KELLY: No.

JANE: Ethnic groups or anything?

KELLY: It's not. Tay-Sachs is.

[It was not necessary to mention another genetic disease at this point. As the next few exchanges show, it resulted in an unproductive sidetrack.]

JANE: What is Tay-Sachs?

KELLY: In Tay-Sachs, the child dies after a few years.

JANE: Is it like they can't breathe in their sleep or something?

KELLY: That's more like cystic fibrosis. Did I answer your question before?

[The genetic counselor does not want to be drawn into a discussion about various genetic diseases, except to point out that there are other genes that have a higher frequency in the population.]

JANE: Yes.

KELLY: I don't feel that you're "beating it."

> [*The genetic counselor's comment about "beating it" refers back to the wife's comment, "And I realize I'm probably beating the thing to death. . . ." (See page 59.)*]

KELLY: (continuing) I think it's something that you've been worried about for a long time.

JANE: Yes.

KELLY: And I think it's hard to give up a worry that you've had for a long time.

> [*The genetic counselor validates Jane's concern.*]

JANE: I'd love to get rid of it. In fact, when I say it deep down feeling like I believe, I think it's true. I think Henry has helped me to feel that I understand systematically the logic behind the statement, "Don't worry about it." For example, the odds of having brown hair among the population of white people must be, what, one to two, must be a big number. That's much harder to understand than what does one in 300 mean. Because I can understand it for a lottery but you can't think of genes in the same way.

HENRY: I think it's kind of an emotional thing because it's easy to explain probabilistic terms like—like I tried to think, "How can I help her?" and I said, "Well, just roughly, what if you went down the street tomorrow and asked the first person you saw today, "Is this your birthday?" That's one out of 365.

> [*Henry hints that emotions are responsible for Jane's incomplete grasp of the probabilities.*]

KELLY: That's ingenious.

HENRY: But that didn't quite go over the same as if you'd say, well, the likelihood that you're going to have severe dandruff is one out of 100 (laughs). But it was interesting, this story about her mother. It's an indication, I think, of how people think about probability because she said over the phone, "Well, the probability of Jane having it was one out of four and the probability of her sister having it was one out of four and so the joint probability that she (the mother) would have two children like that was one out of 16 and that seems like it would be a really small number, and her mother said, "Look, I only had three kids and two of them are like that." So I said to Jane, "Well, let's do an experiment. One out of 16 isn't that small of a number compared to one out of 300, which is much smaller."

KELLY: Yes. That's not quite true though. That doesn't work in genetics.
           Your mother's chance of having a child with albinism every time
           was one out of four.

           [*It is, of course, statistically correct that the chance of having
           two affected children was one out of 16. However, the genetic
           counselor was trying to make the point that each birth (like each
           statistical event) is independent of the event that proceeded it.*]

HENRY: That's right. The chance was one out of four each time the child
           was conceived, but when you look at the whole family, the joint
           probability—it's unlikely for example, if she had 10 kids that
           every one would be an albino.

KELLY: On the other hand, she also had three girls and no boys.

           [*The genetic counselor pursues her point.*]

HENRY: Yes. Yes.

KELLY: Well, you expect 50–50, but we all know families in which there
           are six boys and families where there are six girls.

           [*An example using boys and girls is generally easily understood.*]

JANE: Yes. Yes.

HENRY: Yes. But if you figured the joint probability of say having six
           boys, that's still a high number compared to one out of 300.
           That's what I was trying to get across.

           [*Henry felt comfortable enough with the genetic counselor to
           press his point.*]

KELLY: That's right.

HENRY: Well, anyway, as an experiment, I told Jane to take a nickel and
           we played that the heads were recessive and we flipped coins and
           we got two albino babies. Even though as you say, on each toss,
           it's one out of four and even though it seems unlikely, with a
           relatively small family you can see it done twice. You know there
           are subtleties to interpreting these numbers and I think
           sometimes people can say because their experience showed an
           unfortunate example, that they forget all about all the alternative
           experiences that could counterbalance that.

           [*Henry has given a lot of thought to presenting probabilities in a
           relevant manner and to counteracting his mother-in-law's con-
           cerns. Many people do feel that their own family background
           shows what the "real" risk is.*]

JANE: In fact, I was saying that to Henry. I said that probably in my
           mother's family there are people who have one dominant and one

recessive and the same is probably true in my father's family and they just happened to marry somebody who didn't have an *r* to pass on. And so, of course, everybody else in the whole family is brunette, or all right.

[*Note the equation of brunette with all right.*]

KELLY: I wanted to say. . . .

JANE: What I thought was funny about the numbers is that you start out before you have any children always with a very low probability. Like both of my parents each started out with one in 300 chance. And once it happens, you don't slowly go down in odds, you quickly go to one in four.

[*This is confusing to some people.*]

KELLY: You know why that is, don't you? Because before you're calculating the odds on the probability they each carry the albino gene. Afterward you're very sure about what your parents' genetic make-up is.

JANE: Yes. It would be neat if there were a test and you could know. And they could test Henry and if he had two dominants it would be so nice. It would be more reassuring than probability, even a very very low probability.

KELLY: Of course.

[*The genetic counselor validates Jane's concern.*]

JANE: Because there would be certainty and you really wouldn't have to worry about it.

[*Uncertainty is difficult to handle, even if the probability is low and the disorder is not incapacitating.*]

KELLY: You know, don't you, that the chance that Henry is a carrier is one in 300. The chance that you would have a child who is an albino is one in 600.

HENRY: Yes. Because I might not pass my recessive to you, even if I were a carrier.

KELLY: We really shouldn't talk about one in 300 because you're not really interested in Henry's genes. We're talking about a child right now. The chance that you and Henry together could have an albino child like you is one in 600, not one in 300.

[*The genetic counselor attempts to show that the chance of an albino child is even lower than what the wife might think.*]

JANE: Yes. I thought it was. . . . Are you really sure about that? Or does it go the other way, that it's really one over 150 and then you double it and then it's one out of 300.

[Jane is concerned that arriving at a probability is done arbitrarily. She also seems confused. Therefore, the genetic counselor takes a firm stand in the next statement, while explaining a general rule of probability to Jane.]

KELLY: No! In statistics whenever you use the word *and,* you multiply. So what is the probability that Henry is a carrier *and* he passes on the recessive gene? One over 300 times one-half is one over 600. And I'm positive.

JANE: So far, you've given us two facts of information which are helpful because. . . .

[Here the genetic counselor could have asked what those valuable pieces of information were. In telling them, Jane might have summarized some of the aspects that were most important to her.]

KELLY: Well, that's one reason I had you back because I'm sure Dr. Evans gave you lots and lots of stuff the last time and now you have other questions to ask.

JANE: Well, that's good.

HENRY: I asked Jane when we were coming up here what she wanted to ask, and I think one of the major questions was about getting a feeling for the probability. You know, what other things are there?

JANE: I used an example. I said it's just strange. I don't know about genetic probabilities so it's a strange way to think of it. I used an example. I said, "Suppose somebody had never heard of calories in food. And you tell them a chocolate cake is 500 calories." You don't really appreciate what that is unless you know what other things are. And then you know what a daily average amount of calories is, and then you can appreciate what kind of magnitude you're talking about.

[Jane demonstrates how difficult it is for many people to apply probability to their own lives.]

KELLY: Well, just think back. I think, to get an appreciation—how many children or how many people have you met who are albinos? And you must have been looking much more than Henry or I would, walking down the street.

JANE: Well, I would say in the course of my life, people that I would say, of course, we're not talking about the pink-eyed people because I'm sure they're probably locked up someplace (laughs) in a place where they're cared for 'cause they're blind and they're. . . .

[Jane is very concerned about pink-eyed people. The genetic counselor decides to use an emphatic denial of Jane's perception of albinos.]

KELLY: That's not true!

JANE: It's not?

KELLY: No!

KELLY: There was a beautiful little girl in here not so many months ago. Her parents would be very distressed to hear you say that.

HENRY: I was thinking it sounded a little strong.

JANE: Really?

KELLY: No.

JANE: That's what I'm *afraid* of! I have a scary *impression!*

KELLY: Oh, no. As a matter of fact, sometimes the people with pink eyes. . . .

JANE: If I felt it was a normal thing I could accept, I probably wouldn't have been all upset all this time. You can tell I have a scary impression.

[Jane is now speaking of her deepest concerns—that she might have a child who would have to be "locked up" someplace.]

KELLY: The question with that little girl is whether she is going to be *legally* blind or not. She can definitely see. She's still too young for us to know exactly what her sight is going to be. It's very variable. But she's not ever going to be locked up anywhere.

JANE: I'm sorry. It probably was strong.

KELLY: No. I guess that's your fantasy. And I'm. . . .

JANE: I never talked about it, frankly, but I never saw anybody that extreme. Of course, there's a famous. . . .

[It would have been interesting to hear which famous albino Jane meant. The genetic counselor might have gotten this information by repeating, "A famous . . . ?"]

JANE: (continuing) Perhaps they're a minority group that are kind of badmouthed. You look in very esoteric art books and they always have an albino in the circus. And that is probably the only place I ever saw a true albino. As far as people like me, I've seen about six in my life.

KELLY: Which is more than most people would see. So, it's pretty rare.

HENRY: And again, we're talking about two different problems. I mean. . . .

JANE: I'm talking about people who seem, just on the surface. . . .

KELLY: And some of them might not be albinos; some of them might be just very fair people with flaxen hair. You won't know until you look in their eyes the way Dr. Evans did with you. Okay? Even say six. Let's accept those. So how many people with brown hair have you met?

JANE: Yes.

KELLY: There are just not very many people who are albinos. I think that will give you a good indication of what the carrier frequency is.

[The previous comments are intended to help Jane feel how rare the albino gene is.]

JANE: Yes.

KELLY: Because if it were higher you would see very many more people. It's very rare.

HENRY: Yes.

JANE: Yes. I guess. How many blond people have you seen? I guess maybe 20 percent of the population are blond. Well, if you wonder about that, then, for example, Henry could possibly have a blond child. I'm sure he's got a blond gene in there, but that's a different thing, isn't it?

[Jane wants reassurance that being a blonde and being an albino are different.]

KELLY: Yes.

JANE: Because you're asking about all these weird ones.

KELLY: Weird ones?

[Terms need to be defined. The genetic counselor didn't want Jane to continue to equate albinism with such terms.]

JANE: Rare things in the population; that's why you brought them up.

KELLY: Because we're talking about albinism, which is rare. . . .

JANE: Which is funny because you go to Scandinavia and many people are very tow headed and very blond, maybe 70 percent of the people. I took a picture when I was there because I was amazed. All these little blond kids didn't have an eye problem; they didn't seem to. They looked perfectly fine. Is that a separate gene than the one we're talking about?

KELLY: Yes. It doesn't necessarily mean that they're albinos. The reason I brought up—you said why did I bring up all these weird things—all these rare things? I'm trying to make the point that albinism is very rare and that it is very unlikely that Henry is a carrier.

JANE: I guess what I was thinking was that if he had a gene for blond hair it could all happen. But then that's not at all connected.

[This has evidently been another of Jane's concerns. Note the roundabout way in which the topic was raised.]

KELLY: Not at all. As a matter of fact, I had a son born with blond hair. I have brown hair and so does my son's father. But my son's hair has gotten darker and now he has brown hair. That might happen to you, too. So when your child is born and you see a blond head, if you do, it doesn't mean a thing.

JANE: And their eye color changes too, doesn't it?

KELLY: Caucasian children are born with blue eyes.

JANE: Then they get darker.

KELLY: Some of them do. You might have a blue-eyed child. It's the albinism gene that we're talking about and you have a one in 600 chance of having a child with two albino genes.

[*This is an attempt to clarify the difference between albinism and blond hair with blue eyes.*]

KELLY: (continuing) Would you have said that you have albinism to yourself before you came into the clinic? Is that a term you would have used about yourself?

JANE: No. I'm not really. . . . I wouldn't like to do it excessively either. Because I think it's. . . . I'd put "partial" or something like that in front of it.

KELLY: Yes. That's what I mean.

JANE: No! No! I wouldn't. But. . . . I wouldn't. 'Cause I would have been too defensive.

KELLY: How about now?

JANE: Well, we're doing it. That's all right.

KELLY: But I mean, how does it sound when you say it to yourself? How does it strike you to be labeled?

[*The genetic counselor is probing here to get a better understanding of the impact of the albino label on Jane.*]

JANE: It's not a. . . . It's not a label that I'm particularly proud of.

[*Note Jane's continuing and deep sensitivity to the term albino.*]

JANE: (continuing) In other words, I'm probably not going to *tell* anyone, but I don't feel very depressed or unhappy about it, because I feel that I understand what it really means and that it doesn't really change how I look. By saying it, it doesn't make me see worse or get more sunburned. It's just a word. But, it'll probably take a little more time until I'm really at ease with it. To tell people or to use it freely. Although I was surprised when I wrote that letter to my mother and was trying to be as candid as possible. I did use it. And I was probably more relaxed about using it than I would have been before coming. So that's good. 'Cause I was too emotionally charged up about the whole thing, feeling so defensive and so rare and singled out and odd and victimized by the whole thing.

KELLY: I can see how you might begin to feel that way.

[Jane's response to the disease is acknowledged as a valid one. Then a question is asked to try to assess the impact of genetic counseling.]

KELLY: (continuing) I'm wondering if coming to the Genetics Clinic has changed that in any way?

JANE: Yeah. I think so. I think it's a very good place. It hasn't done me any harm. I've understood myself better. I have probably a better self-image, because our case, of course, worked out better. Maybe for someone who is told something that's not very positive, maybe their self-image changes for the worse. But mine improved, I think.

KELLY: How do you think it helped improve your self-image?

[The genetic counselor asks for specifics.]

JANE: Well, I was told that I'd have a normal baby and that helps. That's a tremendous relief. And what I was told was that what I have is not such a horrible curse that it goes on through your children in a Greek kind of tragedy sense, but that it could stop with me. Which is nice to know, that it's not something I have to feel horribly guilty about. Although I guess I'd always be aware of the fact that the *baby,* the most likely baby, would have a dominant and a recessive and would probably have to be told, "Look, your Mommy's blonde. You probably have this recessive trait. You probably have 10 others that we don't know about, but this one we know about. So you can have that information." Probably won't make any difference to them.

[Jane is again equating blond and albino.]

KELLY: Well, it might even be an advantage because that's one probably, when your baby's older, that we'll be able to test for. And he or she will know to have a test. . . .

JANE: You think they're going to have a test?

KELLY: I'm very optimistic. Yes. Every year there's a new test for something like this.

JANE: Are people working on this particular problem? Do you happen to know?

KELLY: I'm sure they are. Yes. Various aspects of it. The main area of research is how to help increase people's melanin production once they are albinos, to try and turn it on. But what I want to get back to is. . . .

[Changing the subject and checking on the meaning of previous statements.]

KELLY: (continuing) You said something interesting before. I want to see whether I really heard it right. Are you saying that if someone says to you, "You're going to have a normal child," that your self-image is improved? That's an interesting concept to me if that's what you mean.

JANE: Yes. Certainly. Because telling somebody something like that makes them feel happy when they've worried that it was the contrary. It generally changes how I feel. I don't even know if you notice it. I don't even know if it's visible; I guess I feel less horrible responsibility and more—more trust that everything will work out all right with the baby. After seeing Dr. Evans I threw my arms around Henry and I said, "Oh! Great!" What I was fearful about was baby X or feeling a sense of responsibility. I don't want to knowingly harm anyone and also I imagined nine months of sheer hell worrying about this and wondering because of just not knowing.

KELLY: That's a nice story. I'm pleased you brought that up. Henry, have you noticed a difference in Jane?

[The genetic counselor checks with the husband and brings him into the discussion.]

HENRY: Oh sure. She was especially happy the day that we saw Dr. Evans. I was going to say, when you were asking about self-image and all that. When we've talked before, even years ago when we first got married, it was always this kind of feeling that I got from Jane that, "Gee, maybe I can't have a child." Not, not so much that she's physically unable, but she doesn't want to. She's too afraid. And so, therefore that there's something wrong with her. And I think when she realized in her own mind that it was all right for her to have a child, that she didn't have to have this fear, then it seemed that she was okay too. That she didn't have this, this problem. And she was very happy. I think we were both a little amazed when we were talking to the doctor that it all seemed so simple.

[Henry illustrates that people often receive validation from their children—even those that are unborn.]

HENRY: (continues) I thought it had to be a more complex, involved difficult thing. He only talked to us for about five minutes or 10 and. . . . Well, we talked to him longer, but after that period of time, we pretty much found out the heart of the matter.

[Many people worry about the short period of time required for making a diagnosis, and may need reassurance about its accuracy.]

JANE: I guess we kept waiting to hear, "But," and he never did. And I even said that to him. I said, "Aren't you going to say 'but' and tell us the bad news?" And he said, "No, there isn't any."

KELLY: Yes. I had a hard time. I felt fairly sure of the diagnosis during your first visit. There were a couple of times when I said a little bit more than I intended and then backtracked and said, "Well, of course we'll have to look at the chart or wait for the diagnosis.

[*The genetic counselor corroborates the diagnosis made in a previous visit. It is important for counselees to know that the various team members agree with the diagnosis.*]

HENRY: Well, you didn't really give yourself away.

JANE: No.

KELLY: By the way, are you in touch with your married sister?

[*The genetic counselor wants to make sure the sister is told of her real risk, not the risk the mother might think it is.*]

JANE: Yes.

KELLY: Because their chances are one in 1200.

JANE: One over 200 times one-half?

KELLY: Well . . .

JANE: Times one-quarter? What is it?

KELLY: One over 300 times a quarter.

JANE: Oh. I see. Yes.

HENRY: She could have two dominants, right?

KELLY: Right.

HENRY: And then there would be no problem. I mean that's just one of the alternatives.

JANE: Yes. And I think the thing that's confusing to a lay person is when I look at my sister, she has brown hair. I look at her husband and he's *real* dark. It seems impossible. And I think just for my mother, she looks at me and it seems to be impossible, or so unlikely that the baby would be normal *given* I'm the mother, that it shakes her up.

[*Jane is associating phenotype with genotype.*]

KELLY: I gave you the wrong figures for your sister. I'm sorry.

[*The genetic counselor realizes that the risk figure she has given for the nonalbino sister is incorrect and wants to cover the material again.*]

KELLY: (continuing) Let's look at it this way. Your sister's husband has one in 300 chance.

JANE: Right.

HENRY: Your sister has a two out of three chance of carrying the recessive.

[The married sister has a two out of three chance of being a carrier of the recessive and a one out of three chance of not carrying the recessive.]

KELLY: That's right, $^2/_3 \times ^1/_4$.

HENRY: Yes.

[At this point the genetic counselor has started writing down the important figures and labeling them so the couple can see the figures as she refers to them:
    $^1/_{300}$ chance husband is a carrier of the albino gene.
    $^2/_3$ chance the sister is a carrier of the albino gene.
    $^1/_4$ chance the sister and her husband will have an albino child, if they are both carriers of the albino gene.
Their risk of an albino child is therefore: $^1/_{300} \times ^2/_3 \times ^1/_4 = ^1/_{1800}$.]

KELLY: That's her husband's chance ($^1/_{300}$). Your sister's chance (two-thirds) times putting those two together (one-quarter) to get the child. So that comes to 900 times four, 3600 to one over 1800. That's the chance for your married sister.

HENRY: As compared to, say, normal of one over 300. Or one over 30,000 for the general population, so they definitely have a higher chance than the general population, but lower than us, which you'd expect.

KELLY: One over 1800 is not anything to get really. . . .

JANE: You know, my sister and I never really talked about it. I don't know if she is afraid or isn't afraid, or knows anything about the particular difficulty or not.

HENRY: I might say that both Jane and I expected her mother to be very happy and very excited about what we learned in genetic counseling. Because certainly *we* were. We wanted to tell them not because we thought they had to know, but because it would be fun to tell people, people close to you. I was very surprised to hear her mother react with anything less than enthusiasm. Then after Jane told me about the call, I started to realize that at least on a rational plane her mother didn't seem to be able to appreciate the differences in the two situations. . . .

JANE: I think she felt that Henry's and my chances were *much* higher than hers and my father's chances. Of course, when I figure out that ours were 82 times better, that even surprised me because I had never thought of it that way. I figured it out. I did the percentages. Their percentage of risk is 25 percent. Ours is 0.3 percent. So the magnitude is a lot different.

[*Here the wife is talking about the* 1/300 *or 0.3 percent chance that her husband is a carrier. However, their chance of having an albino child, as mentioned earlier, is calculated as follows:*

1/300 *chance the husband is a carrier of the albino gene.*

1 chance the wife is a carrier of the albino gene.

1/2 *chance this couple will have an albino child if the husband is a carrier of the albino gene.*

$1/300 \times 1 \times 1/2 = 1/600 = 0.16$ *percent.*]

KELLY: Remember last time we were talking and I asked you what risk would be acceptable? Remember what you said?

[*The genetic counselor decides not to return to the* 1/600 *figure given Jane earlier, but to reenforce the concept that 0.3 percent is, indeed, a low risk figure. The 0.16 percent is brought to Jane's attention later.*]

JANE: I said 5 percent.

KELLY: Yes. Then you said maybe less than 10 percent. But now we're talking about 0.3 percent. And, Henry, you equivocated. You said, "Well, if we really want children in the future, 50–50, I guess." But really you said you'd like something like 10 percent.

[*The couple is reminded that the present risk they face is smaller than the risk they had previously said was acceptable.*]

HENRY: I remember I was willing to give more.

KELLY: So now we're talking about 0.3 percent as opposed to that.

JANE: And someday they're going to have the test. It'll either be 0.3 or 0. It's tempting to want to have a definite answer 'cause the probability is great. I mean by that, it's wonderful.

[*The wife wishes the uncertainty of probability was not present. Note the variety of ways in which the word great can be interpreted.*]

JANE: (continuing) I guess you just have to learn to live with it. Life isn't so well-ordered that you can *know* things. There are unknowable things I guess.

KELLY: Any time you have a child you never know. The birth of a healthy child is really a miraculous, beautiful thing. And, of course, you know, even your 0.3 percent is not really concerned with an unhealthy child.

[*The genetic counselor tries to show that every prospective parent faces uncertainty.*]

JANE: No. It's sort of assuming something. And I guess you shouldn't. You should be grateful for it more—in awe. It is miraculous. I agree with you.

KELLY: Yes. I'm not trying to play it down. I'm just saying that if worst comes to worst, again your worst fears are not going to be met, in that you're not going to have a pink-eyed child that has to be locked up. I think all mothers or mothers-to-be have some sort of fantasy like that.

[Jane's concerns and fears are validated.]

HENRY: That kind of relates to something that I sort of wanted to ask about the clinic. Maybe this is interesting to you too because you seem to be interested in some of the human ramifications of some of the things that you're doing.

I was a little embarrassed to come here with all this apparently high-powered consultation: a group of doctors, and you, and a medical doctor and several visits for what seemed to me, although I knew it meant a lot to Jane and it was a problem, a small problem compared to some of the other problems that are genetic and that you may have to talk to people about.

[Often counselees are reluctant to ask for help, since they feel they may be taking up time needed for others who have more serious concerns.]

HENRY: (continuing) You talk about something like cystic fibrosis or even sickle cell anemia. And I wonder how you see that. Well, you've talked about seeing others like this couple with an albino baby and apparently following the literature, so albinism is enough of a problem that people do keep up with it. But, was my feeling justified to an extent? Does it seem to be one of the very mild problems on the spectrum of what is a proper topic for the clinic? Or is this maybe my own hang-up about whether we really have something important enough to warrant this much discussion?

KELLY: Yes. I'm wondering where it comes from. When you go to the doctor with a really bad sore throat or something, are you one of these people who has a nagging worry that it will disappear just as soon as you get inside the doctor's office?

HENRY: No. I think it was more a feeling that there are probably a lot of people who need the services more, who don't have access to this clinic or anything like it, and I wondered if we were taking advantage of the fact that we knew enough to look for things like this and we could afford, not so much this clinic, but just regular and adequate medical care that can lead you to a clinic like this.

KELLY: I see what you mean. We consider everybody with whom we make an appointment seriously and make appointments with people that we *can* consider seriously. Because by the time people get to us, they're highly motivated and they're concerned and it's a happy day for us when we can give people good news. Sometimes people come who have absolutely nothing wrong with them genetically, just nothing. They're concerned that they might and that's fine too. So we consider their concern a legitimate

problem to bring for genetic counseling. It's nicer to deal with
something like this than people who just had a baby die, or people
who have a child born with mental retardation. That's a heavier
thing. But we take this just as seriously.

JANE: (continuing) We were quite impressed with the attention that we
got here. The explanations were so clear. I think that the clarity is
helpful even if it's bad news. You want it. People want it, I'm
sure.

*[Time and again people ask for clarity and information, saying
that it is the unknown that is scary.]*

KELLY: We do try and give it clearly, as clearly as we can. I like to give
the whole story. A lot of people are worried as you were that we
will leave out the "but." That we try very hard not to do, but to
be very honest with people. Then they can make up their own
minds.

*[The genetic counselor again assures the couple that they have
heard all the information that is available.]*

KELLY: (continuing) You know, if you two decide that one over 600 is
much too high a risk to take, we can sit back and say, "Well,
okay." We'll try and give you the figures in such a way that you
will understand it well. We feel good when we've given complete
information; then the responsibility goes to you, and
appropriately so.

*[The genetic counselor wants Henry and Jane to hear again that
decisions are theirs to make, and that $\frac{1}{600}$ is the correct risk
figure.]*

KELLY: You talked about your family. What about friends? Have any of
them been told?

[One topic is ended and another started.]

HENRY: I haven't told any of them.

JANE: I guess I haven't, although I almost did. There are some people
that just seem very sympathetic. I think partly I didn't really have
a close enough friend out here that I would share it with.

KELLY: I wonder if there are any parts of the counseling that are still
unclear, that you'd like to get straightened out.

*[Before closing the session, the genetic counselor checks to see if
there are any unanswered questions.]*

HENRY: Not from me. I think everybody's been very patient and helpful
as far as answering every possible question that we can think of.

JANE: That we can think of.

KELLY: I have no more questions to ask. I want to thank you both for coming, for sharing with me what happened.

[The conversation continues for some time after the genetic counselor has officially ended the session. It is not uncommon for counselees to discover that they have a lot to say just as the session ends. For this reason the wise genetic counselor "ends" early.]

HENRY: Oh, it's kind of fun.

JANE: It's nice for us too because it sort of finishes it all out.

HENRY: Also, with Jane's discussion with her mother in the last few days, new kinds of questions have cropped up. And you helped us with that too.

JANE: Sure. Definitely. So perhaps this second visit had more use than we thought it would. It *was* sort of forced on us. But I'm glad we did it, because things did come up. And we did think about it some more.

[When this couple learned that there was a routine follow-up visit, they were initially uninterested, and said that they might not have the time to return for it. They were told that such visits were routine, and that we would like to schedule one and hope that, as the time drew near, they would find the time to attend.]

HENRY: After we saw Dr. Evans, I don't think we had any questions, but it was nice to wait a couple of weeks and then discuss things.

JANE: I think it's nice too, because I'm sure people think up their own questions or talk to their friends or their family and they say, "but." And I'm sure this visit helps reemphasize facts that might have been forgotten when they were talking to their uncle and he said, "but." It's a strange interplay of emotional and medical, factual things. And I'm glad you realized you can't do one without the other. You can't just give people the cold facts and you can't just say, "Oh well, you're okay. Don't worry. You pass our screening." And you give them some score. They want to know as much as possible about the medical information and they also want to feel like the person is understanding how they feel or aware that they're afraid or that they're glad. So I think it's all very good.

[Jane has eloquently summarized some of the reasons for having follow-up visits.]

KELLY: I'm pleased it was helpful. You know how to get in touch with us if you come up with any more "buts" or any more questions.

[Jane and Henry are assured of continuing help and support by the genetic counselor.]

HENRY: We have your little card with everybody's name on it.

[A card with the names and telephone numbers of genetic clinic staff members was given to Jane and Henry during a previous visit.]

JANE: So. We're all done.

HENRY: Yes.

KELLY: Good night.

JANE AND HENRY: Good night.

[Since both Jane and Henry work this visit was held in the early evening.]

6 Emotional and Social Reactions to Genetic Disease

> Health is not a state of being; it is a process of adaptation to the changing demands of living and the changing meanings we give to life itself.
>
> D. Mechanic, 1966

Known genetic diseases are numerous (2336 according to the 1975 edition of McKusick's catalog), ranging over virtually every clinical category, and varying from those whose impact is relatively minor (such as brachydatyly) to the very severe (e.g., osteogenesis imperfecta). Sometimes the disease afflicting them is already well known by individuals who seek genetic counseling since they or their relatives may have had the disease for some time (e.g., Marfan's syndrome). At other times, individuals may be in the process of learning about the disease for the first time during genetic counseling, since their child may have just been diagnosed as having the disease or problem (e.g., Down's syndrome or Tay-Sachs). Therefore, the genetic counselor can expect to encounter a wide range of reactions to genetic disease, depending on the situation, the severity of the disease, and when individuals learned of the problem. Yet the counselor will also note some fundamental similarities of reaction in most cases, since genetic diseases raise a question about individuals' capacities to produce a normal child, or even about the worth of oneself.

Stigma   Individuals who seek genetic counseling sometimes have a physical handicap or abnormality themselves, and may be touchy about references to or questions about their problem. They may feel stigmatized, either that they are not as good as others, or that others (the "normals") believe that they are not as good. Individuals may feel stigmatized not only when they have a disease that is visible to others (e.g., albinism), but even when the difference is known only to themselves (e.g., presence of chromosome translocation). In consequence, withdrawal from others, shame, depression, loss of self-esteem, self-hatred, and the use of the stigma as an excuse for all of life's adversities may occur (Goffman, 1963; Geis, 1972). The genetic counselor can be on touchy territory very quickly with someone who feels stigmatized. Such a person may interpret information as an insult, and questions as prying. As Goffman (1963) notes: " . . . advice to the stigmatized often deals quite candidly with the part of his life that he feels is most private and shameful . . ."

For those with visible defects, Macgregor (1970) has suggested that predictability of response to a deformity may be of more importance than the severity of the visual impact. That is, individuals with more noticeable anomalies may become accustomed to reactions of shock or surprise. Those with more "marginal" anomalies may suffer more because they are continually uncertain of their reception by others. One woman sought genetic counseling for Marfan's syndrome. As she left, she commented that she had felt comfortable this time talking about her physical symptoms. She hesitated, then said:

> But someone could look at me strangely this afternoon or tomorrow someplace else and my feelings could be hurt anytime because of it. It makes me very nervous. I never do know what's going to happen.

Individuals who do not have a genetic disorder themselves, but who are related to someone with such a disorder may bear what Goffman calls a "courtesy stigma" (Goffman, 1963). As described by Birenbaum (1970):

> They are "normal" yet "different." Their normality is obvious in their performance of conventional social roles; their differentness is occasionally manifested by their association with the stigmatized during encounters with normals, from conversations that barely skirt certain topics or clumsily touch upon these sensitive subjects.

Such individuals may deny their affiliation with the affected person, maintaining that they are completely normal. Others may throw in their lots with the affected person and consequently become labeled as different themselves. Still others take a normal stance at one time and an affected one at another. Birenbaum (1970) in a study of 103 mothers of mentally retarded children found that these mothers minimized the differences between their families and "normal" families, but maintained their distances from normal families as well. Less than half the mothers in the study had directly told friends and relatives that their children were retarded.

It is not uncommon for parents of children with a birth defect to relate a growing feeling of estrangement from their friends. Some parents, to maintain the illusion of being "just like any other family" report they have not told most friends and associates of their children's diagnosis. One couple who did tell a pregnant friend, learned that the friend was advised by her mother to stay away from them and their child lest she miscarry!

Chronic Sorrow

According to Olshansky (1962), most parents of retarded children suffer from "chronic sorrow" that lasts a lifetime, and is a normal reaction to their child's retardation. Other reactions of parents of mentally retarded children are anxiety, guilt, denial, and hostility toward the doctor who made the diagnosis (Solomons and Menolascino, 1968). One study showed that of 67 families with a mentally retarded child, nearly one-third rejected the diagnosis of mental retardation after the initial diagnosis and workup (Graliker et al., 1959).

When a handicapped child is born, it has been suggested that parents mourn for the loss of the normal, expected baby. At the same time, they must attempt to meet the needs of the affected child (Solnit and Stark, 1961). As Cohen (1962) notes, the added stress of a handicapped child can be most difficult for the family to handle. The effects of a retarded child on the normal siblings include anxiety, guilt, and anger (San Martino and Newman, 1974). Carr and Oppé (1971) have found that the birth of a handicapped child damages the self-esteem and confidence of the parents in their own eyes and in those of their relatives. Mothers of congenitally handicapped children have been found to feel that their own imperfections were responsible for the child's handicap (Tisza and Gumpertz, 1962). Other reported reactions discussed in an informative review by Freeman (1971) include denial, preoccupation with practical problems, dissension between parents, religious conflicts, and fear of further pregnancies.

In coping with the death of an infant or child, parents have been found to go through the three stages of mourning described by Lindemann (1944): shock and disbelief, developing awareness of the death, and resolving the loss. Immediate reactions on the part of the parents include loss of appetite and insomnia (Klaus and Kennell, 1970). Sexual feelings are also often either diminished or absent (Macintyre, 1975).

Some of the reactions to genetic disease most commonly encountered in genetic counseling sessions are discussed below.

Anger Couples whose child has died, or who have recently learned of a genetic disease are often angry. Many do not know how to cope with this strong emotion. One father said: "What am I going to do with my anger? Who am I going to take it out on?" A deeply religious woman whose child had Down's syndrome said: "I get angry a lot. I really do. I get angry at myself. I think I get angry mostly with God. Because I think that we can ask questions, but we get no answers from Him. It's hard." Another woman, who had recently been diagnosed as having epilepsy, reported:

> I feel a little bit against the wall by suddenly being told, after a whole life of being pretty healthy, "Well, you're going to have to take this the rest of your life. Maybe your kid will too." You have tremendous anger and there's nothing you can do with it. There's no way of getting rid of it and there's no way of bottling it up.

Guilt Individuals frequently express guilt about the genetic disease in their family. Parents often verbalize the belief that they might have caused their child's abnormality somehow. For example, one mother reported:

> The thought of genetic counseling just terrified me. I really feel responsible. There's a lot of guilt and that's what keeps you from coming in. It might be confirmed, "Yes, it was something I did."

Many parents continually cast about in their memories, looking for some incident to fasten on as "the cause" of their child's disease or problem. A woman whose child had Pierre Robin syndrome decided the cause must have been an X ray of her wrist she had had when she was pregnant. She said:

It's just irrational, but I didn't want the X ray, you know. And then
of course, you look for things. After the child is born, you go
backward and think of what may have happened during the
pregnancy. You cannot really put your finger on anything, but I
suppose anything's better than nothing.

A father whose child was mentally retarded expressed the
concern that he might have been the cause of his child's
abnormalities "The other thing is, I worked in hospitals as
an X ray technician. So there's a possibility that maybe it's
in my chemistry. I'm just trying to find out."

Other parents have suggested that their child's problem
might have been caused by events that occurred during
conception, such as a lightning storm, or during pregnancy: a car accident, drinking too much soda, "a pill to
stay awake," or an argument. A woman whose retarded
son had not thrived after birth felt his poor health might
have been due to an illness she had had during pregnancy
when she ate very little for a week. Usually such specula-
tions are raised in a cautious, embarrassed manner with an
apologetic laugh, sometimes not until the second or third
genetic counseling visit. Most parents openly express
relief when the genetic counselor takes these fears seriously and explores them with the family. In some cases, it
is possible to show couples that the events of concern
could not possibly have caused the problem, thereby further relieving their anxiety and guilt. In other cases, especially when the diagnosis is uncertain, parents may prefer
to believe that they have determined the cause of their
child's problem, perhaps, as suggested by Bard and Dyk
(1956), in an attempt to gain mastery in the face of
disorder.

The sense of guilt often extends to siblings, and even
cousins, of individuals with genetic problems, though with
them the guilt may take quite a different form from that
expressed by parents: "It isn't at all simple what I feel
about my sister's retardation. I feel awful. I feel in a way I
was so lucky to be me and not to be her. Maybe that
implies a little guilt, too."

At genetic counseling sessions people may even be
heard to express guilt over the emotions engendered in
them by their problem, such as sadness, despondency, and
lack of sexual feelings. Some wonder if they are normal or
"losing my mind a little" with worry or concern, and
express guilt at not being able to handle the situation with

less intense emotions. Many individuals express relief when they are reassured that their reactions are normal.

Poor Self-Image   It is not uncommon for people to make self-deprecating remarks during genetic counseling sessions and to reflect a poor self-image. One woman with a mentally retarded brother reported she had felt: "There's something wrong with me that isn't right, that no one can see, but it's really there." When she later learned that her brother's mental retardation was due to a birth injury rather than a genetic defect, she reported: "I started looking at my hands and saying, "Wow! All these cells are O.K. I'm not defective!"'

Another woman who had Marfan's syndrome said:

> I'm always amazed when I see myself in the mirror and see how big my hands are. I'm not aware of them being especially large until I look in a mirror or see myself brushing my hair off my face in a store window and I can't believe how big they are. I think, "Oh, how gimpy!" But what do you do? Walk around with your hands rolled up all the time?

This woman, as well as others with poor self-image, reported difficulty relating to friends and family. In most cases a feeling of being different is given as the cause of the difficulty with others. Whatever the cause, people with poor self-image are often reluctant to seek comfort or advice from friends and extended family members.

Blame   In an attempt to find a cause for a birth defect, one spouse sometimes blames the other, or a parent will report that he or she had been blamed by a relative. The father of a mentally retarded child said: "But wait! One thing we haven't mentioned is that when my wife was pregnant, she was strangely sick. You were nauseated for six months or so, weren't you?" His wife denied that she was sick that long. Her husband persisted:

> The baby used to have a big belly. I saw a picture of one of these starving kids that reminded me of her an awful lot. So I have a feeling in one way or another she may have been affected by malnutrition before she was born.

Blaming, or the fear of being blamed, sometimes keeps individuals from asking questions they consider important. Whether parents blame each other explicitly or in a veiled manner, it is important for the genetic counselor to try to keep communication between the parents open and direct. (See Chapter 7 on Genetic Counseling Techniques.)

Embarrassment During genetic counseling, individuals sometimes speak of the embarrassment caused by their own or their affected relative's physical problem. A woman whose brother had Down's syndrome said:

> It is very difficult with a child like that, especially when you bring him out in public. He's embarrassing to you, but you're even more embarrassed for him, because he has all the difficulties and there's nothing you can do to right the wrong. It's very maddening because you just want to shake him good so everything will fall back in place and he'll be O.K.

Feelings of Selfishness In some cases, individuals' first reaction to the thought of their anticipated genetic counseling session was that they felt selfish. In these cases, the rationale was usually that, "It would be putting our relatives to too much trouble to get all those medical records." In several instances, it took years for individuals to face the prospect of asking relatives for information. One woman, who was concerned about Huntington's disease in her father's family related what happened when she told her mother she would like her father to get an examination:

> Lately my mother's been acting like she doesn't want to know if he has Huntington's disease or not. Because I was talking to her. I guess I was being selfish in my own way. I was trying to explain to her that if Dad went and found out if he had it, it would help my husband and me a lot—just kind of prepare ourselves for whatever is going to happen. Plus our families too, you know. And she just said, "Well, maybe *you* would like to know because you would like to plan a family. But why put a person in his grave 10 years before it's going to happen?"

In another case a man was most apologetic about his "selfishness" in taking up the genetic counselor's time for such an "insignificant" problem. He had juvenile onset diabetes.

Fear of Genetic Counseling For some individuals there is a two- to five-year interval between the decision to seek genetic counseling and the actual call for an appointment. People delay a genetic counseling appointment for many reasons, among them fear about what they might be told, denial that there is a problem, or embarrassment. For example, a woman whose son had Waardenburg syndrome described what happened when she called for genetic counseling:

> I've had the genetics clinic number taped up above the phone ever since Dr. Ash gave it to me. When I called I was given the idea that it was a total kind of genetic survey, so I canceled the appointment. I dismissed the idea of genetic counseling after I canceled the appointment. Never talked about it to anyone. I got to talking to my therapist and he said that it appeared to him that I was very worried about it. The more we talked about it the more it appeared to me also that I was very worried about it. And that closing my eyes and not making the appointment or having canceled it didn't make it go away. Not knowing was really worrying me.

Another person said:

> I waited I guess three months before I got myself together enough to speak to my mother about it. I had to talk to my mother about it, which wasn't that easy, in order to get her to sign a release to get the medical records sent on my sister.

Denial   Denial can take any number of forms in genetic counseling, some of them quite extreme. Counselees may feel that the genetic counselor doesn't know what he or she is talking about, that the disease isn't as serious as the counselor suggests, that the child will grow out of the problem, that the tests have been misinterpreted, etc. Sometimes individuals feel they have been misdiagnosed since the genetic counselor's description of the disease does not perfectly fit all members of their family.

An attitude some individuals express is that of minimizing the seriousness of the disease in themselves and in their own families. This can be unrealistic and thus a form of denial, but such an attitude can also make it possible for the individuals to carry on bravely or cheerfully despite the burden of their affliction. A man with Alport's syndrome said:

> I can live with kidney conditions and renal failure because transplantation is getting to be, certainly not an everyday occurrence, but by the time our children would be old enough, with the progress that's being made, the picture looks very bright. But I would feel very bad bringing a child into the world that had a physical handicap that would never go away—that they would have to live with and would be apparent to everyone. I think maybe it's vanity.

In many instances counselees deny on one level while accepting information on another. Obviously, if counselees denied completely, they would not seek genetic counseling. In my experience, most denial expressed in genetic counseling has a wishful or hopeful quality. Individuals who deny in one session frequently feel less need to do so in subsequent visits. Also, individuals frequently express both denial and acceptance in the same session. For example, a young father whose infant son had Down's syndrome denied that there was anything wrong with his son. In the same session he expressed keen interest in enrichment activities for his child, such as an Early Infant Stimulation program. Instead of confronting this father with his contradictory statements and obvious denial, the genetic counselor acknowledged the man's desire to do all that he could for his son, and recognized that, like many parents, he wanted his son to excell. In later counseling sessions, this father proudly told how much more his son could do "than most Down's kids."

Individuals may at first deny a diagnosis that suddenly changes their self-image in a way that they had not anticipated. How the counselor introduces new information can affect greatly the tenacity with which the individual will cling to denial. One woman came for genetic counseling because of "hypertension" in her family. In taking the pedigree and examining medical records, the genetic counselor found that the woman had "blackout spells" which she had attributed to hypertension. The genetic counselor made the diagnosis of esoteric migraine and abruptly told the woman that she was not hypertensive. At first, in part due to the way in which she was given the new diagnosis, the woman refused to believe it:

> I'm still adjusting to being hypertensive and he tells me its migraine. Psychologically you don't suddenly become a labeled person. The effect of his (the genetic counselor) saying that it's esoteric migraine and could very easily produce children with migraine, possibly with my sort of complications, was totally off the wall to me.

In a later counseling session, some of this woman's reasons for denial became more clear. She said: "Maybe there's still part of me that wants to be told, not only your kid's not going to have it, you're not going to have it either.'' In handling this sort of denial, the genetic counselor needs to work slowly and patiently with the client. The woman with esoteric migraine was far more receptive to the diagnosis when the way in which the diagnosis was made was carefully explained to her. Even then, she needed several months to become adjusted to the new label.

Many mental health professionals maintain that some form of denial almost always occurs when an individual faces a new or crisis situation and that it may be an essential part of the process human beings work through in order finally to adjust or cope. (See Aguilera and Messick, 1974 and Parad, 1965 for readings in crisis intervention.) The genetic counselor, therefore, must proceed with subtlety in dealing with denial. The counselor need not feel duty-bound to strip away without delay all of the family's illusions about their situation. It may prove more fruitful to explore with the family that part of their denial that blocks understanding of the genetic counseling information. In this way, successful genetic counseling can be achieved without undermining the family's coping processes.

Coping   In much of this chapter and throughout this book, the difficulties and problems encountered by genetic counselors have been raised and discussed. It would be erroneous to give the impression that genetic counselors deal only with individuals who are unwilling or unable to confront their situation. Even when the genetic disease is quite severe, genetic counselors will find individuals who fully and realistically grasp the implications of the disease and cope heroically with their problems. Without minimizing the pain caused by their disease, some may say that their suffering has helped them to grow. A woman whose grandmother, mother, and sister all had Huntington's disease said:

> And I think once you're in a situation, it isn't as drastic as it might be if you were an outsider looking in, thinking, "My God, how do they cope with this?" You're in it, so you do what you have to do. There have been hard times. I'm not saying there haven't been. And it's been very upsetting in many areas and experiences. But all in all it's helped build character in me too. And it's given us a real closeness.

Another woman whose four children had retinitis pigmentosa wanted her children to be studied, not just for their own benefit, but for that of others:

> I think it's something that I as a parent can contribute to a child that may be born in later years with this same problem. It may help another parent face some of the things that they're not able to face. Or better, know what they can look forward to.

7 Genetic Counseling Techniques

One gains knowledge when information is broken down and assimilated into the personality. Until this is done, information is like a tool which is useless because the person doesn't know how to handle it. Learning is not simply a matter of acquiring information. The learned person knows how to apply this information to life, especially to his own life. He has related it to his feelings and has integrated it with his experience.

A. Lowen, 1970

Genetic counseling is a hybrid field, utilizing a combination of knowledge about medical genetics and counseling techniques. Just as genetic counseling may be imprecise without reliable diagnostic capabilities, it can be ineffective without adequate counseling skills. Because genetic counseling is a relatively new field, its counseling techniques are still being evolved. Many of the techniques and practices now used have been borrowed from psychology and interviewing. Families are often involved in genetic counseling, so a knowledge of family dynamics and how to counsel families is needed, as are techniques from crisis intervention for individuals who are in a crisis state.

Care must be taken in adapting techniques from other fields for use in genetic counseling situations. Obviously, most counselees will not be in a crisis state. Many may not be overly or unduly alarmed. Individuals who seek genetic counseling, unlike individuals who seek family or crisis counseling, have not come for help with an emotional problem, but for help with a genetic or potential genetic problem. While it is self-evident that many genetic diseases can cause tremendous social and emotional strains on families and individuals, the focus of genetic counseling is to help individuals to understand the genetics of the disease so they can reach decisions that are appropriate for them. To this end, counseling skills are needed to elicit from individuals their perception of the problem and its causes and to communicate effectively about the disease and its genetic aspects in a way that is meaningful to the individuals seeking counseling. In addition, a complete genetic counseling service provides referral to appropriate social services (e.g., early infant stimulation programs for infants with Down's syndrome, or to other appropriate forms of counseling (e.g., family therapy).

Throughout the genetic counseling process, the emphasis should be on clear communication. To achieve this communication while dealing with sophisticated technical information and the emotional and social problems often caused by genetic disorders is the genetic counselor's challenge. For convenience, the following discussion of techniques has been divided into: considerations before the first session, opening the session, the body of the interview, and closing the interview, as well as specific approaches to counseling.

Considerations Before the First Session

Making the Appointment

Counseling techniques need to be employed even before the genetic counselor and family meet face to face. When an individual calls for an appointment, he or she does so with certain concerns and expectations. Many prospective clients are nervous. They are apt to be sensitive to how the first telephone call is handled. For example, one woman canceled her first counseling appointment. During a subsequent one she told me she had come "determined not to let you make me into a weirdo." She said that when the receptionist had asked on the phone "the nature of your birth defect" she had become defensive and had replied that she didn't have one. According to this woman, the receptionist then asked, "Well, if you don't have a birth defect, why do you want to come here?" Obviously it is necessary for the secretary or receptionist to ask those who phone for an appointment the nature of the concern or problem, since without such information the genetic counselor cannot schedule properly. Yet the secretary or receptionist should be aware that many people feel awkward or embarrassed about their problems and should be trained to elicit the needed information tactfully.

In another instance, a woman whose son had developmental problems canceled her genetic counseling session when she was told over the phone by the receptionist that she and her husband should come prepared to discuss their own and their families' medical histories. "I thought they were trying to pin the blame on us," she explained. Nearly a year passed before, with the aid of her psychiatrist, she could bring herself to reschedule her counseling session. In this case, the receptionist either did not have the time to explain why the records were needed, or did not sense that the woman viewed the request for medical records as a threat. Misunderstandings of this sort can be avoided if the need for the records is immediately explained.

The Environment

As mentioned in Chapter 2, the environment in which a counseling session occurs also affects the nature of the sessions. *Every effort should be made to provide a room that is conducive to open and direct communication.* An appropriate counseling room is one that is private, cheerful, comfortable, and free from distracting noises. Privacy is essential, since many genetic counseling sessions deal with intimate matters. Even a private room is insufficient if loud and distracting noises occur nearby. Most disturbing, as has been said, can be the sound of babies crying to people whose child is sick or who has recently died. Many genetic clinics are crowded, and examining rooms are used for counseling sessions. In such cases, it is important that the genetic counselor not overwhelm the family by sitting on the examining table and looking down upon them. Rather the counselor and family should be able to sit facing each other, on the same level.

The social environment is also of importance. Parents often cannot concentrate on what the genetic counselor is saying or remember questions they wished to ask if they have a whimpering baby on one knee and a toddler actively exploring the waste paper basket. Supervised child care needs to be provided for children, so the parents can give their full attention to the counselor. The child must be near the counselor's office so the children can be examined and (when appropriate) included in the counseling itself.

The genetic counseling environment should also include

charts, blackboards, and perhaps, slides. The easy accessibility of these educational aids increases the likelihood that they will be used and indicates to the family that these aids are an integral part of genetic counseling, not special equipment brought in for less intelligent people.

Opening the Session

The first few minutes of a genetic counseling session do much to shape the rest of the hour. The family immediately notes and reacts to whether the genetic counselor is on time or is late; is rushed or unhurried in greeting them; looks concerned, sympathetic, stern, or judgmental. Starting immediately with the introductions, the genetic counselor can model direct communication by clearly identifying him or herself and his or her role in the genetic counseling process. Each member of the family can be greeted unhurriedly to demonstrate that the counselor has time for, and is interested in each individual. Time spent defining relationships, obtaining proper pronunciation of names, and discovering the preferred method of address can gracefully bridge the first few moments and set the tone for the rest of the interview. By taking time with introductions, the genetic counselor is saying nonverbally, "This is a place where there is time for each of you to speak and to be heard." In addition, a warm welcome can do much to make people feel comfortable in what, to them, is probably an alien environment.

One way to relieve their initial anxiety is to provide the family with information about the counseling service's procedures and personnel. Sometimes people may need information about the physical setting, or the relationship of the physician to the hospital or laboratory. For example, if the genetic counseling service is in the pediatrics department, some adults will wonder if the clinic can provide information about genetic diseases in adults. In addition to being informative, this type of general conversation gives the family a chance to size up the genetic counselor and begin to feel more at ease.

If the counselor and family have not spoken previously, the counselor can ask how the family learned about genetic counseling: Who told them? What have they been told about that particular counseling service? Such a discussion enables the counselor and family to get used to one another, and indicates some of the family's past experiences and present expectations. From this initial exchange, the counselor begins to gain an understanding of the family and its concerns.

The Body of the Interview   In the first session, the genetic counselor will want to learn why the family made an appointment for genetic counseling and what they expect to gain from genetic counseling. For example, one man with a mentally retarded brother said:

> Well, what I was expecting was a chromosomal pattern test just to see if there were any deformities or any absences that would indicate certain diseases. A sperm count would have to be checked to find out whether the sperm itself is of insufficient count or is deformed.

In previous attempts to get genetic counseling, no one had asked this man what he expected. He had never been told that neither karyotype nor sperm counts were needed, so he had continued to seek new sources of counseling. Information about expectations is best obtained from family members in person, even if the counselor has had previous discussions with the referring physician or earlier telephone contact with the family. By making sure that each family member has an opportunity to respond, the genetic counselor can learn about differences in individual approaches, expectations, and reactions, without acting like an inquisitor, and can also gain a sense of the dynamics of the family involved (e.g., who speaks first, who interrupts whom, and who answers what). Sometimes the concerns expressed will be different from those the counselor anticipated. For example, one father of a mentally retarded son was interested in the prognosis and possible treatment of his affected child. He had several normal children and was not planning to have more children. "It's really a birth defects thing that we're interested in. I don't know if we're interested in the genetics."

By encouraging the family to talk at the beginning of the session, the genetic counselor can quickly learn the family's assumptions about the nature or seriousness of the disease. Without an understanding of the individual's view of the disease, the counselor may later present information in a way that will shock, numb, or lead to denial. One man with a retarded son told how he felt after receiving information about his son's condition:

> When you're beat up and somebody comes along and kicks you, you know, is it gonna hurt? You're already lying on the ground, beat up. You're not gonna feel one more. That's about it. That's the way I feel.

Much of the body of the interview flows naturally from, and is dependent on the family's opening statement. In the first session, the family as well as the counselor will have many questions or matters they would like clarified. Concerns range from specific questions about causality, as expressed by a young father whose infant had died: ''Who can really cause it? Me or her? Would it be in the sperm, or what?'' to a desire to know more about whether a future child will be affected and what might be involved in the decision to plan a family: ''We've been mulling this over for about a year—whether we should or shouldn't have children. Now we can plan our lives instead of having this up in the air hanging over our heads.'' In the intake visit, there is rarely enough information to give specific answers. However, concerns can be acknowledged by the counselor and assurance given that concerns will be discussed at a future time when more information is available.

Usually, in the first visit, the genetic counselor elicits the history of the disease in the family and how family members have reacted to the disease. In subsequent sessions, the counselor explores individuals' reactions to the new information they are receiving. One way to do this is to alternate questions about fact with those of feeling or affect. For example, after being told what an individual learned in a previous session, the genetic counselor might ask, ''And how did you feel about that?'' or ''And that information made you think? . . .'' or ''So the effect of hearing such and such was? . . .''

In subsequent sessions, the genetic counselor can learn much about the ongoing concerns of the family at that point by asking at the beginning of the session such questions as, ''How have things been since I last saw you?'' or ''What's been happening since we last spoke? How have you been feeling about the information you received last time? What have been your thoughts about the information you received last time?'' The family can then bring up issues and questions which are of relevance to them at that time.

It is important to discuss issues that the family may raise before going on to issues that the genetic counselor feels are important, since individuals can be given information many times, but usually hear or really understand this information only when they are ready. Thus the counselor should recognize the family's agenda and respond to it.

The genetic counselor also needs his or her own agenda for each counseling session, since without such an agenda, the counseling session may wander aimlessly. The initial interview will generally include such topics as decision and procedure (how and when the decision to seek genetic counseling was made), expectations (about genetic counseling and the risk of disease recurrence), the family's genetic history and psychosocial reactions to the disease, and family history (medical, genetic, and social). Subsequent interviews will depend on the family's responses during the initial interview and the genetic counselor's understanding and assessment of the problem and concerns. In general, future visits will include discussion of such topics as what individuals learned during preceding visits and the impact of the information on their lives. (For the types of areas to be covered in initial and follow-up visits, see Appendix A.)

By having an agenda in mind, the genetic counselor can remember to return to areas that might otherwise get cursory treatment or be neglected altogether. To ensure that certain areas are covered, the counselor may want to refer to a questionnaire or checklist during the session and say, "An area I want to cover today is. . . ." If a topic has not been covered to his or her satisfaction, the counselor can raise it again, saying, "I want to explore . . . at greater length," or "I'm not sure I fully understand what you said about. . . ." At some point, the counselor may want to look at the list for a minute or so to make sure all areas have been well covered. Again, a direct statement about the activity can be made. Initially, genetic counselors sometimes feel embarrassed if they have to look at a list or if a lull in the conversation develops. However, a pause can give people much-needed time to reflect.

With experience, counselors become more adept at linking their own and the family's agendas. Rather than having many breaks between topics, experienced counselors are able to blend one area into another in the course of the discussion. However, in many sessions, the counselor may want to abruptly change the subject in order to end a monologue by a monopolizing individual, to encourage a shy individual to talk, or to cover an important topic before the end of the session.

Closing the Interview

In all likelihood, the genetic counselor has told individuals about how long their session will last that day, so the impending end of a visit does not come as a surprise, and is less likely to be taken as a rejection. Ten to 15 minutes before the end of a session, it is often useful for the counselor to announce that the time is almost up. (A clock on the wall that is visible to both counselor and family generally produces less anxiety in the family than a watch the family cannot see, but that the counselor is frequently checking.) When the end of a session is announced, many people suddenly remember issues they want to discuss. By "ending" early, the genetic counselor allows time for these issues to be raised. It is more important for issues to be raised than that they be discussed immediately. After acknowledging that he or she has understood the new issues, the counselor can defer them until the next session.

Near the end of the session, the genetic counselor may want to ask the family how they feel about the areas that have been discussed, and what issues they would like to discuss further during subsequent sessions. Individuals then have an opportunity to summarize, for themselves, what has occurred during the session and to note issues that need further resolution. The counselor may also summarize, emphasizing both the points that have been covered and those that are still unresolved. At this time the counselor can suggest areas for further thought by the family.

In some cases, the genetic counselor may want to reassure an anxious family that they have come to an appropriate place and that they will be given complete information when it is available. For example, the counselor might say:

> I know your major questions are . . . and . . . I'm going to speak to Dr. Roth, who is a specialist in this area. When you see her next week, she will have read your chart, the most recent medical articles, and spoken with me about your problem. Be sure to take your questions with you. Write them down if you think you might forget them. After your visit with Dr. Roth we can discuss the implications of what she has said.

Such a statement shows the family that the genetic counselor will continue to help them, even though another specialist is needed. It helps allay any uncertainty they may have that they won't understand the specialist, since the genetic counselor will be available for future discussions. Such reassurance often helps individuals learn more from the specialist than they would have thought possible.

A closing summary by counselor and family leads naturally to a discussion of the next session, its date, and its purpose. By discussing a specific date and time for the next session, people are given concrete proof of the counselor's continuing interest in them. As with the opening, the closing of an interview takes time. Farewells can begin with the counselor expressing a complimentary (and sincere) statement to the family. This helps even those who have had a sad interview (e.g., "It seems to me that throughout the last few months you have been a very courageous family. I'm impressed."). Although a friendly and personal parting with each individual in a family is important, it is sometimes difficult to achieve this with people who are embarrassed or shy. In such cases, the genetic counselor may have to cut short goodbyes with some family members to ensure that others do not slip away.

Most counseling sessions take about one hour. When possible, sessions should be scheduled at least one and one-half hours apart to allow for families who need more time, and for individuals who may be late. This extra time can also be used by the counselor for writing notes about a completed session, preparing for the next session, and relaxing. Since genetic counseling can be emotionally draining for the counselor as well as the family, a counselor often needs time between sessions to unwind.

Specific Approaches to Counseling

Acute Listening and Observation

Most genetic counselors think it is their job to talk knowledgeably—to transmit information. However, they need also to listen. Listening well takes a special talent. Listening means not just keeping quiet occasionally to allow the counselee to talk, but actually putting all one's attention and awareness on what the speaker is saying. By focusing attention on the speaker, a greater understanding of what the problem means to the person becomes possible. People being counseled often drop hints of areas they would like to discuss but are unsure of how to raise directly. By listening intently the genetic counselor is more likely to hear the hints and can introduce the topic for discussion.

Listening intently and watching carefully also help the counselor decide on the most comprehensible manner in which to present genetic information to the family and how he or she can help the family work through its emotional reactions to the disease and to genetic counseling. An astute counselor will watch and listen for inconsistencies in the medical and social history, inappropriate comments or gestures, and repetition of patterns that can block communication. By gently pointing out an inconsistency (e.g., an individual denying, then acknowledging that he is a sickle cell carrier), the genetic counselor can help individuals become aware of issues that they are avoiding. Inappropriate comments or affect (e.g., laughing where one would expect sadness) show the counselor areas with which the individual has not yet been able to cope. In one case, a woman who had epilepsy said: "And the fear of being there and dying on my own, was being very bad to me." (laughs) In such cases the counselor may say, "I notice that when you talk about . . . you laugh." At other times the counselor may note these areas and discuss them directly or obliquely at a later time or not at all. In many cases, the counselor may note inconsistencies or denial, but not point them out, if to do so would embarrass the individual or hinder understanding.

A perceptive genetic counselor looks for signs of nonverbal communication. Exchanged glances between family members, body posture, a scowling face—all convey meaning. Sometimes the counselor will note but not comment that an individual looks disturbed when a particular topic is raised. The counselor may want to raise the topic at a later time or mention what a painful area it can be. At other times, the counselor may want to ask what a particular look means or if the individual has noticed that she scowls when a topic is raised. Body language can also give the counselor important clues about the individuals being counseled. Do they lean forward anxiously to catch every word (or is there a hearing problem)? Do they sit with arms and legs tightly folded as if frightened (or is it too cold in the room)? Are they too shy to meet the counselor's eye, (or is there a cultural prohibition against looking directly at the counselor)?

The intently listening counselor can learn much from sighs, words spoken too low to be heard, sentences that are not completed, and the quality of a person's voice. As with other observations, the counselor must carefully decide when these signs should be mentioned and when their discussion would be painful or pointless. Generally in counseling involving fewer visits, the genetic counselor must be more cautious because he or she will have less information on which to base observations and less time to deal with individuals' reactions to these observations.

Sounds. Often people are not aware that they have sighed or giggled. By bringing such observations to their attention, the counselor can give them an opportunity to discover the meaning of these sounds for themselves. There is obviously a difference between making the observation and interpreting the meaning or significance of the observation. The latter is best left to the individual or family.

Inaudible words. When the genetic counselor cannot hear words or sentences, it is important that he or she ask the person to repeat them. Often these words are of great significance, but the individual is not sure how they will be received by the counselor or other family members. Sometimes complaints are presented in this fashion. An alert genetic counselor will note such drops in voice level and immediately ask for clarification, thereby demonstrating respect for the individual, and his or her thoughts and feelings.

Incomplete sentences. Communication is often enriched when individuals are encouraged to finish their own sentences. Genetic counselors can help in this process by repeating the last spoken words and ending with a questioning inflection. People are most likely to leave sentences unfinished when they are unsure how to end them. For example, one father said, "When we got to the hospital I kept trying to ask. . . ." When he was encouraged to finish the sentence he realized he had not asked the doctors anything, because he did not know where to start. It then became apparent to him that he had been having the same trouble formulating questions in the genetic counseling session. In some cases, it is helpful for individuals to try different endings to see how each feels. For example, a prospective parent who has just said, "Well, a 25 percent chance sounds like a, a, you know," can try saying, "A 25 percent chance sounds too risky to me," and "A 25 percent chance doesn't seem all that high." Discussion about how each of these endings sounds and feels is often helpful to individuals.

Tonal quality. Voice quality can give clues about the speaker's current emotional state. For example, a metallic or monotonous quality might mean that the person is depressed. An individual who speaks softly may be shy or embarrassed. Tonal quality, like other nonverbal signs, is a clue to be used in conjunction with other evidence. Unless the counselor is cautious in interpreting such signs, individuals may be classified too rigidly by the counselor.

Family Processes

Patterns of behavior are important to a genetic counselor, since they provide information about the ways in which the family functions. For example, families differ in the ways they reach decisions. In one family a mother of a child with Waardenburg's syndrome made known her desire to have no more children by dropping hints offhandedly. Her husband then pronounced that same view as the family's decision. Subsequently, the wife acceded to "his" decision. The genetic counselor who is unaware of this family's decision-making process can become entangled in defending either the downtrodden wife or husband, depending on the perspective. The real point, however, is that a family *process* is involved, requiring the active participation of both members of a couple. If the wife in the example just given later complains that "my husband makes all the decisions," the genetic counselor who has recognized the pattern will be better prepared to help her become aware of the role she played in making the decision. In short, an understanding of a family's patterns enables the genetic counselor to help the family reach decisions that are acceptable to all family members, and decreases the likelihood that the genetic counselor will be caught in the family's process, or used by one family member against another. (For books on family therapy, see Haley and Hoffman, 1967 and Satir, 1967).

Listening for Relevance

It sometimes happens that genetic counselors find themselves losing interest in a topic being discussed. Instead of trying to listen harder, the counselor may find it useful to try to discover why his or her interest is flagging. For example, is the client talking about an area that he or she thinks will interest or impress the counselor but is of no interest to him or her personally? To check this out, the counselor might ask the client if this is a topic that is of real interest to him or her at the moment. Sometimes clients will say that they are no longer sure why they are talking about that particular topic. The counselor can then help the individual think back to what brought the topic to mind in the first place. Often the individual has an important piece of information to tell, but has gotten sidetracked. If the individual states that the topic is of relevance, the counselor can either ask for clarification or listen for a few more minutes to see if the area then ties in with other issues. In some cases, the counselor may want to indicate that the topic has been covered sufficiently for his or her purposes, and to ask if the individual would feel comfortable going on to another area.

Sometimes individuals talk animatedly or with strong emotion about a topic that does not appear relevant to the counselor. When this occurs, the topic usually has a relevance which the counselor does not yet see. In some cases, the relevance will become apparent later. In others, the counselor may want to ask, "And the connection between your sister's child with diabetes and Down's syndrome is? . . ."When a seemingly irrelevant concern is explored, it can lead to another concern that has relevance (e.g., the parents fear that having diabetes in the family will increase their risk of having a Down's child). An apparently irrelevant monologue may be what some people use to test the genetic counselor to see if they can safely raise the more troubling issues lurking below the surface.

Asking Questions

Although most people derive considerable relief from being able to express their emotions and to speak at length to the genetic counselor, the genetic counselor may need at times to interrupt what they are saying to gain more information about a particular point or to make sure he or she has understood what the family is saying. Individuals who are encouraged to continue their story following an interruption, or point of clarification, rarely feel the counselor is not interested.

As noted earlier, the family may have concerns about the disease that are completely different from those that the genetic counselor assumes they have. To learn what people want from their counseling session, the counselor must often ask them directly or ask if he or she has correctly understood what is wanted. In many cases, family members are unsure of what they want or of what they can get from genetic counseling. Once the family's uncertainty has been acknowledged, counselor and family can work together to define and, as counseling continues, redefine what the family wants from genetic counseling. By redefining the family's goals at different stages, the counselor can help the family to see counseling as a process, and can validate individuals' changing thoughts and feelings throughout it. In fact, if genetic counseling is succeeding, the family's concerns *should* change, since they will be gaining new information and new perspectives on the relationship of the disease to themselves.

By asking people what they think and feel about past events pertaining to the disease and information given during genetic counseling, the genetic counselor models direct communication for the family and for family–genetic counselor interactions. The counselor does not assume an omnipotent stance toward individuals' feelings or knowledge, nor does the counselor assume that people will think or feel the same way throughout genetic counseling.

Summarizing and Checking

Words have different meanings for different people. For this reason, it is essential for the counselor to summarize what he or she thinks an individual has said, and to ask the client if this understanding is accurate. Sometimes the counselor has incorrectly or imprecisely understood the meaning of an individual's words. By repeating the essence of the message the counselor enables the individual to correct and to refine the impression the words have made. Not only does the counselor understand the intended meaning better, but counselees are helped to think about the meaning of their own words. Until individuals hear the counselor's summary, they may be unaware of how their own words had sounded. Individuals may not even be aware of inconsistencies or the depth of the feelings they have projected.

A summary of the communication also demonstrates to individuals that the genetic counselor is really trying to understand their positions. Sometimes people repeat themselves until the counselor demonstrates this understanding by accurately summarizing what the individuals have said. If the counselor does not try to change an individual's opinions or feelings, but attempts to gain an accurate understanding of them, a person will speak of thoughts, beliefs, and feelings without fear of being judged. Often, when there is no resistance to a thought or to an opinion, people will reverse their positions in a short period of time. The genetic counselor's role at such times is to help individuals to understand the implications of their current thoughts and beliefs, leaving the evaluation of various alternatives to the counselees.

Counseling Stance

Inherent in the term genetic *"counseling"* are the somewhat different connotations of consideration, contemplation, reflection, and deliberation on the one hand and advice, opinion, recommendation, and suggestion on the other. Which of these two directions is the genetic counselor to take? Is the genetic counselor's task one of leading clients to the "right" decision, based on his or her knowledge of medicine and genetics? Or is the genetic counselor's task one of presenting "just the facts" in a nonpartisan manner? Obviously, the latter course is never completely possible, since the genetic counselor will have his or her own opinions and feelings which will be expressed in nonverbal, if not verbal, ways. The issue really is the *degree* to which the genetic counselor should try to influence individuals' decisions.

While it is true that genetic counselors know more genetics and medicine than their clients, and have had more experience with the implications of various decisions, it would be a mistake to conclude that they also know what a "better" or "right" decision would be for a particular family. People vary greatly in their approach to illness. For example, as discussed in Chapter 8, socioeconomic status and ethnic origin affect how often and when different people will seek medical care (Koos, 1954; Zola, 1963a), as well as their perception and interpretation of symptoms (Zborowski, 1952). It is hardly surprising that their reproductive decisions should vary as well.

The genetic counselor can best help individuals reach a decision by creating an atmosphere in which people feel comfortable examining an issue from many different perspectives. By listening to what may appear to be irrational and nonscientific beliefs about a situation, the genetic counselor demonstrates respect for the search individuals are undertaking. Out of this unhindered search often come more satisfying solutions than are possible when individuals feel constrained to find or recognize the "right" or "reasonable" path.

A neutral counseling stance is not usually possible if the genetic counselor has strong feelings about what the family should or should not do (e.g., abort an affected child). When the counselor disagrees with the family's decision (or projected decision), or can comfortably contemplate only one decision, he or she can either have someone else counsel the family or else carefully examine his or her own assumptions and their underlying value structure. It may become apparent to the counselor that his or her disagreement with the family's decision cannot be resolved by logical discussion, but arises from a conflict of basic values. The genetic counselor's task then becomes one of making certain that the family's decision is in accord with its own values.

Alternatively, when the genetic counselor has been able to pinpoint the basis of his or her uneasiness with the family's decision, it may become apparent that the counselor's and family's basic values do not differ in this area. By suggesting that a contradiction exists between the family's stated values and its decision, the counselor may assist the family to further clarify its own thinking. In some cases, the decision will be reversed. In others, as in the case of a man with Alport's syndrome, people will acknowledge that their decision is not entirely rational, but is due to their overwhelming desire to have children "anyway." As this man said:

> I felt there would be some people who would say, "Well, the simple solution is not to have any children." That's the obvious solution. And that we are being selfish to pursue the matter to the point of going to genetic counseling. Why do we really want to have children, given the nature of our risk involved? Maybe since there is a risk of some sort at all we should just say, "Let's not have children." That would really be the noble or the rational thing to do. I felt a sense of guilt almost in pursuing the chances as far as we have. I felt a sense of guilt until I got to the point of thinking, "Well, damn it, why does anyone want to have children?" It's a selfish thing in a sense. And we have a right to pursue it.

This man, like others, was fully informed about the risk to future children and the nature and consequences of Alport's syndrome. Further, he and his wife had fully considered at length how their lives would be affected by having a child with Alport's syndrome, combined with any further medical problems the man might have. The genetic counselor's task had been completed. This does not mean that the counselor personally would have made the same decision as that couple, but that the decision was seen as the couple's, not the counselor's, right and responsibility.

There is some disagreement among genetic counselors themselves about the burden of different genetic diseases. Some feel that having a child with kidney disease or mental retardation would place the most stress on a family, while others feel that a more visible disease such as neurofibromatosis could present greater problems. In one study (Sorenson, 1973) genetic counselors were asked about the burden of various diseases on an affected individual. Of the almost 500 respondents, five percent thought diabetes mellitus was very serious, 31 percent serious, 47 percent moderately serious, 15 percent not too serious, and two percent minor. In the case of Down's syndrome, 65 percent ranked it very serious, 25 percent serious, seven percent moderately serious, and two percent not too serious. Hemophilia was ranked 41 percent very serious, 45 percent serious, 13 percent moderately serious, and one percent not too serious. By becoming aware of the diseases that cause him or her more unease, each counselor can guard against overreacting to those diseases. It is not necessary to stop counseling for such diseases, but rather to become aware of one's own feelings and biases. Such an awareness enables the counselor to effectively help different families with the same genetic disorder make entirely different reproductive decisions— and to recognize that these decisions may be perfectly "right" for each family. There is no one standard for judging the seriousness of a disease, or the correctness of a decision. For this reason, each family must make its own decision, based on its life values and emotional tolerance.

If a family looks to a genetic counselor to make a decision for them or to assess the impact of a given affected child on their lives, the counselor can say, "I think you are wanting me to tell you what decision to make or what I would do in your place. It's very tempting for me to do just that. After all, I do have thoughts and feelings about what I would do. But you are the people who have to live with the decision, not me. If you make a decision just because I'm comfortable with it, that won't help you in future years. Now, let's try to figure out what I can tell you to help make a decision that fits you." In such a safe environment, many people will "try on" various approaches, attitudes, and solutions, using the genetic counselor as a mirror to see how these new attitudes fit. Instead of spending energy convincing the genetic counselor that a given thought, decision, or approach is appropriate, individuals can concentrate on how different decisions would fit into their own lives and value systems.

Being a Catalyst

A catalyst is a substance which can speed up a chemical reaction but is not itself permanently changed or bound to other reactants. The genetic counselor, like a catalyst, can speed up the family's coping and decision-making processes by helping the family work through the informational and emotional issues which relate to the genetic disease. Just as a catalyst is not permanently bound in the reaction it accelerates, the wise genetic counselor avoids being bound up in the family's interactions. By being available to facilitate communication and give information, while leaving the responsibility for decision-making in the hands of the family, the genetic counselor:

1. Reaffirms his or her confidence in the family's ability to solve its problems;
2. Avoids becoming entangled in family disputes or taking sides;
3. Maintains enough objectivity to give the family a fresh perspective, but is there to support and help if needed;
4. Avoids a situation in which the family waits for the genetic counselor to make a decision for them.

Instead of being placed in a dependent role, the family is respected as coequal with the genetic counselor. Therefore, counselees do not need to be helpless or incapacitated to receive the genetic counselor's help. As Chapter 8 shows, parents who are placed in a dependent role may lose their self-esteem as parents, and thereby become less capable in that role.

8 Sociological Aspects of Genetic Counseling

Illness behavior and the decision to seek medical advice frequently involve, from the patient's point of view, a rational attempt to make sense of his problem and cope with it within the limits of his intelligence and his social and cultural understandings, but this does not make it rational from a medical perspective.

D. Mechanic, 1968

The role of the family and the role of children in the family have undergone many changes in the last few centuries. Families have separated themselves from the society around them, with the nuclear rather than the extended family becoming the predominant type. Even within the last 20 years the structure of the American family has undergone great changes. The number of children per family has decreased, the divorce rate has increased, and married women are increasingly likely to work outside the home.* Changes in family structure have resulted in a smaller familial network from which individuals can draw help and support during times of illness. Instead, individuals must rely to a greater degree than ever before on social networks outside the family: friends, social service agencies, medical institutions, and health professionals.

As more children have survived childhood, and as the ideal (and actual) number of children in a family have diminished, more energy and attention are given to each child. According to M. E. Goodman, "We have set a new

*For interesting discussions of the implications of these recent changes, as well as an historical perspective, see Ariès, 1962; Skolnick, 1973; de Mause, 1974.

record; no other people seems to have been so preoccu-
pied with children, so anxious about them, or so uncertain
about how to deal with them," (as quoted in Skolnick
1973, p. 314). Skolnick suggests that as local communities
have diminished in importance, people turned to their
families for social sustenance. However, with decreasing
family size, there are fewer people to whom an individual
can turn in time of trouble. In a genetic counseling session,
one man responded bitterly when asked what his relatives'
reactions had been to the death of his infant son:

> They wouldn't care. They don't want to talk about family
> problems. Everybody's back East and that's good. They have their
> own healthy children and nobody is really interested. It's just between
> us two.

People without close friendships or family ties may feel
particularly vulnerable to the stresses caused by many
genetic diseases. Therefore, the genetic counselor will
want to quickly ascertain the support systems available to
individuals. Ironically, as extended families have diminished in number, so have general and family practitioners
who traditionally knew an individual's whole family and
way of life, and who could offer a meaningful kind of
emotional support. According to Kendall (1971), the
remaining general practitioners see an average of 21.9
patients a day, a number which "would hardly permit
them to provide care at a leisurely pace." Obviously,
individuals who have little familial, social, or medical
support may need greater support from the genetic
counselor.

Within our own pluralistic society, individuals vary
greatly in their concept of family and the need for children
in the family. For example, some individuals seeking
genetic counseling come from more traditional families,
with close ties to extended family members. Others are
from nuclear families and have few, if any, ties to
extended family. Regardless of the family background,
individuals frequently need help from the genetic counselor to clarify what children mean in their lives, and what
sacrifices and chances they are willing to take to have
future children. From the multiplicity of possible feelings
about children, family life, and coping with disease within
the family, individuals who seek genetic counseling make
choices that best meet their frequently conflicting needs as
parents, individuals, and spouses. As this chapter shows,

sociocultural factors play a large role in determining individuals' reactions to children and family, health and disease, and other matters pertinent to genetic counseling.
Individuals are usually not aware of the implications of
these underlying cultural attitudes. Part of the function of
the genetic counselor is to be aware that sociocultural
differences exist, and to help counselees become aware of
the issues involved in making reproductive decisions that
are appropriate to them.

In making a decision about whether to have a child,
prospective parents who seek genetic counseling balance
their need and desire for a "normal" child with their
perceptions of the risk and the consequences of having an
affected child. In so doing, they show a variety of ways of
viewing prospective children. Sometimes the same person
will have several different perspectives simultaneously.

Some people are unsure about whether they want to
have children until they learn what the risk of having a
child with a genetic problem might be:

I don't even know if and when or anything I want to have a child,
but I thought perhaps one reason that I don't know is because maybe
in the back of my mind I do feel there is a chance that I'd have a
retarded child as my mother did.

A woman with Charcot-Marie-Tooth disease put her feelings even more strongly: "I think my feeling is that I'd be
god-damned if I want a kid to go through that." The
husband in another couple whose child had congenital
cataracts said: "We weren't about to commit ourselves
and our emotions to wanting—to admitting we want children if we knew that there was a strong possibility there
was no hope without a terrible chance."

For some people, the decision about whether to have a
child seemed to depend on how the child would later view
the affliction, should she or he have it. Some counselees
expressed concern about what the prospective child would
think of them "to take a chance like that," while others
said they would not feel guilty about having a child with a
birth defect if they had done all they could to prevent such
an occurrence beforehand. Still others felt they wanted to
be prepared for such a child: "I just think the fairest thing
to a child being born is to know what to expect."

Many prospective parents said that their desire for
children fluctuated with time, as did the risk they were
willing to take. One woman with neurofibromatosis said:

> We don't really want children for the near future, so we can perhaps be very choosy and say, "Well, the risk has got to be really low." But if we really want to have a child anyway, I think something like a 50–50 chance would be it.

Other people saw the fluctuation in willingness to take risk as a function of energy available to cope with an affected child: "If I felt I had the strength to deal with a child that would need a lot more energy from me, a high risk would be all right."

Not surprisingly, individuals with a genetic disease sometimes feel that they would not want their future child to have that disease. Individuals with a dominant genetic disorder sometimes feel that although the effects of the disease on their life has not been serious, the same gene might produce more serious consequences in a future child. Since many dominant disorders vary in expressivity, this is a realistic concern. In one family, the wife very much wanted to have a child. The husband, who had Ehlers-Danlos syndrome, did not want to take the risk of having an affected child. He said:

> If the child is affected, it will take much more energy from me. I'll have to deal with all the hospital business, all the specialized surgery, all the specialized needs. Having gone through that myself, I don't want to take the chance that I'll be as good a parent as my parents were in the sense of knowing how to deal with that situation. And maybe my kid won't come out as well-balanced as I have. Maybe he'll come out bitter, as a lot of people who have handicaps are.

Since the husband realized his wife wanted a child very much, he expressed concern for his wife's wishes, while continuing to believe that they should not have a child:

> It gets really difficult for me. 'Cause, you know, it's my love for you in wanting to give you something that feels really dear to you. My love gets in there and my reasoning process gets really screwed around. Part of me says, "Go ahead and have a child," and then the other part says, "If you do that you're going to be sorry."

In this case, husband and wife were approaching a consensus of opinion (that the risk of having a child was too high for them), but had not yet reached it.

Some individuals with genetic disease feel strongly committed to having a child. They feel that since the disease has not been severe enough to limit their enjoyment of life, it would not be onerous to future children.

When one woman with juvenile onset diabetes was asked what an acceptable risk figure would be, she said:

> I don't follow percentages too closely. I guess I'm more of a fatalist. When something happens I face it. In other words, I'm not that concerned about the situation. But I am interested in knowing what there is to know.

Later in the visit, it became apparent that she did not want to consider juvenile onset diabetes as a serious disorder:

> But the thing is, having lived with the disease for that long a time, I feel in a fairly confident position to say how I feel. I don't think it's complicated my life and I think I've led a good life to this point. That's why I'm not so overzealous about just picking a percentage and deciding one way or the other.

Since she had the disease, she did not want to think that its consequences could be grave. Therefore, she claimed not to be interested in the risk figures that could be provided by genetic counseling. A man with Alport's syndrome who had decided to have children before he sought genetic counseling felt that neither the risk nor consequence to future children would be serious:

> Well, my reservation was that since we were going to bear a child in any case, and the chances of its being severely deformed were probably small or hard to predict, that I wasn't exactly sure what the role of genetics counseling was.

Sometimes people seeking counseling feel they can handle some problems but not others in a child:

> I think that we're both willing to deal with certain types of genetic defects. Like, neither of us has very good eyesight. If a child of ours were nearsighted, as it very well might be, this would be passable. On the other hand, there are certain things that we really wouldn't wnat to risk if there was any substantial probability of it. Like Mongolism, any kind of really serious deformity, kinds of hereditary blood disease, schizophrenia.

Some people with genetic disease want to have a child to show that they are as whole and as normal as others. Some want to have "a child like me." Others have weighed the seriousness of the disease and their desire for a child, and have found the desire for a child to be stronger. For example, the man with Alport's syndrome quoted in the previous chapter said: "And I don't mean to say what I have is not bad, to brush it aside. What I'm saying is that it's not severe enough given the sense of want for a child."

For some people, the wish to have a child is so strong that they may have difficulty hearing information about the possibility of having an affected child. For example, some people seem to have made a decision to have children before seeking genetic counseling and hope to get facts to buttress their decision. A man with neurofibromatosis commented:

> Should we even seriously consider having children since there is a health hazard? Coming to the genetic clinic for counseling was a pretty self-motivating thing looking for someone to tell us that it wasn't so bad.

Prospective parents who have been told that their offspring might be affected rationalize their decision to take a risk in a variety of ways. Some point out that since no prospective parents can be given a guarantee that their offspring will be healthy, they might as well take a risk also, even if it is somewhat larger: "If you carry the argument to its logical extreme, you might say that there's practically no one who's justified in having a child because there's always that possibility of a really tragic outcome." A man who was contemplating a consanguineous marriage said: "And we do have reasons for wanting to have a child which, I think, are as valid as anybody's."

For some people, children are a continuation of themselves or of their family. For others, children are seen as the way to create a new family. Still others look to children for company. One woman whose husband had a genetic disorder that could shorten his life said:

> And then I get little selfish feelings of what am I going to do if my husband dies early and I'm left all by myself? I'm not close to my family. And there I'd be. Who would have me? No one would have me at age 55. I would be too young to die and too old to get started again. I don't know. There's that fear of being left. I'd like to have the security of family around.

As mentioned in Chapter 6, one common reaction parents may have to giving birth to a child with a genetic problem is a loss of self-esteem. Individuals who believe themselves to be at risk of having a child with a birth defect, as well as identified carriers of genetic disease, may suffer from a lack of self-esteem, even if there are no affected children. One woman who learned she was a carrier for Tay-Sachs disease said: "It's not like anybody else. It's genetic. It's hidden. It's not something you can see, but it's there." This woman felt that since she might some day have an affected child, she was in some way affected herself. Another woman whose sister was retarded said: "I thought that I too was defective and it just didn't show so much on me." As described in Chapter 6, when the woman learned that her brother's mental retardation was not of genetic origin, she no longer felt "defective." Still another woman, whose follow-up visit is reported in Chapter 5, related that when she realized that there was very little chance that she would have an albino child, her own self-image improved. None of these women had had an affected child, yet all had had their self-image and self-esteem lowered when they thought that a future child *might* be affected. These examples indicate that not only present, but future children can play a role in shaping an individual's self-esteem.

There are undoubtedly many complex factors and emotions that go into individuals' feelings about children. As one man said: "You don't really decide that you want or don't want to have children. That's not a decision. That's a feeling." In a few visits, the genetic counselor cannot hope to sort out the reasoning and emotions behind individuals' views on children. However, if counselors are aware that individuals differ in their approaches to children and family life, they will be able to help prospective parents gain more insight into their own thoughts and feelings. Such insights can help individuals assess their genetic risks from a fresh perspective and increase the chances that individuals will make reproductive decisions that are suitable to their needs.

Individuals differ in their views about and reactions to illness as well as to families and children. In recent years, studies in medical sociology and anthropology have been concerned with the social and cultural aspects of reactions to illness, how medical care systems are organized, and the ways in which medical care is delivered. From these studies, it becomes apparent that there is no one correct or normal response to disease or to the threat of disease. The fear, disgust, stigma, or indifference associated with a given disease varies with individuals and with their cultural and social background. For example, as is shown in Chapter 6, some individuals are more concerned about mental retardation, while others are worried about a visible physical deformity. One woman said: "We didn't tell people that the baby was deformed. We just said she had heart problems and left it at that. I think people can tend to get morbid about it." To this woman, a heart problem was an acceptable problem, while visible, external abnormalities were not. Unfortunately, many discussions on genetic counseling have focused on "how to tell the patient" or "when to tell the father," as if one standard explanation or procedure would apply in all situations.

From medical anthropology and sociology, genetic counselors can obtain a general framework in which to consider genetic counseling issues, as well as learn how different kinds of people approach and respond to illness. These disciplines can also provide insight into some of the communication problems that can exist in interactions between counselees and health care professionals, thereby helping genetic counselors to view their counseling situations with increased objectivity, and providing new clues for communicating with individuals who seek genetic counseling.

In this chapter, some of the findings of medical anthropology and sociology most relevant to genetic counseling are discussed in three main areas: reactions of patients or clients, doctor–patient communication, and reactions of physicians. For more readings in this area, see Mechanic, 1968; Freeman et al., 1972; Jaco, 1972.

Reactions of Patients or Clients

Use of Medical Facilities

In general, individuals with higher socioeconomic status and higher educational levels are more frequent users of health care systems (Anderson and Andersen, 1972). This greater use is probably linked to an increased perception of need for medical care (Koos, 1954), and greater knowledge about specific diseases (Samora et al., 1962), as well, of course, as greater ability to afford such care.

One study has shown that 13 percent of all people who seek genetic counseling do so before the birth of an affected child (Sorenson, 1972). These cases can clearly be classified as preventive care—individuals' attempts to prevent or detect disease in an asymptomatic state (Coburn and Pope, 1974). However, there are individuals who have an affected child and *then* seek genetic counseling, and relatives of affected individuals are also often interested in preventive care. Therefore, much genetic counseling is probably of a preventive nature.

The most important indicator for determining who will seek preventive care has been found to be high socioeconomic status (Coburn and Pope, 1974). It is therefore likely that people who seek preventive genetic counseling frequently come from upper socioeconomic levels. A knowledge of socioeconomic level can be helpful in assessing individuals' reactions and behavior during genetic counseling. For example, individuals with greater economic resources can more easily pay for the extra housekeeping, babysitting, special tutoring, or physical therapy that might be required for a child with a physical or mental problem. One man, whose wife was a carrier for hemophilia said:

> My feeling is I don't really want to mortgage away the rest of my life to a male child. To have that kind of financial liability. I think of it in terms of having to make that much more money. It would change my life.

Cultural (Ethnic) Background

Individuals from different cultures perceive health and illness differently. For example, in the Mexican-American culture, individuals are assumed to be healthy if there are no overt symptoms of disease (Abril, 1975). Therefore, in the absence of overt symptoms, some individuals may have difficulty accepting a diagnosis or understanding the desirability of preventive care. Also, individuals may have beliefs about causation that differ from those of traditional medicine. In the Mexican-American culture, for example, congenital malformations and mental retardation may be attributed to misbehavior on the part of an individual or are seen as a sign of God's displeasure. Exposure to lunar eclipse is thought by some to cause cleft lip or palate (Abril, 1975).

Such beliefs may be stronger than people may admit at first, even in supposedly sophisticated societies. Individuals' beliefs about causation are not always readily apparent. Some people may be embarrassed to even mention what they consider the "real" causes of their child's disease (e.g., an argument, careless exposure to the moon, drinking soda, a moral transgression). Part of the genetic counselor's role is to explain the transmission of the genetic disorder, if it is known. Unless an individual understands such an explanation, he or she can leave genetic counseling still clinging to the old belief. Therefore, the genetic counselor must spend some time learning each individual's belief about the cause of the disease, as well as the reasoning or belief system that led the individual to hold the belief. It will not always be possible to convince individuals to give up their misassumptions, even when these are contrary to scientific evidence, but a genetic counselor who has established rapport has a better chance of doing so than a counselor who hasn't. One woman believed the reason her child had Down's syndrome was because she had taken a pill a friend had given her to help her stay awake during the night shift at the factory where she worked. She had taken the pill during her fifth month of pregnancy and "didn't feel right" for the remainder of the pregnancy. Although she and her husband had been told that Down's syndrome was the result of the presence of an extra chromosome in their child that was present from the time of conception, she had not put the two facts together. When the genetic counselor pointed out the discrepancy, a pleased look spread over the woman's face. She could stop blaming herself as she had been doing.

Individuals from different cultural backgrounds may manifest symptoms differently and have different concerns about similar symptoms. In a classic study on cultural differences in response to pain, Zborowski (1952) found that Jews and Italians tended to be expressive and emotional about pain, while those of "Old American" European extraction usually expressed little emotion about their pain. The three ethnic groups had different responses to pain as well: "Old Americans" expressed confidence in the future and scientific cures; Italians were concerned about the immediacy of the pain and felt comfortable taking medicines to relieve pain; Jews were concerned with the symptomatic meaning of the pain to their future health, and worried about taking medicines. Genetic counselors need to be aware that what they might consider an excessive display of emotion or an inappropriate lack of emotion can be culturally based. In one couple whose child was stillborn, the husband, of Scandinavian background, seemed unconcerned and unmoved. During a genetic counseling session, his wife, who was of Italian extraction, accused him of not caring and threatened to leave him. He responded that her "excessive" show of emotion was useless and embarrassing to him. In the discussion which followed, the genetic counselor was able to help both members of the couple see that they each cared, and were each responding in accordance with their different family backgrounds. In subsequent discussions, both were able to ask questions about genetics, without fear that they would blame or be blamed. The wife, in particular, had many questions that hadn't seemed pertinent previously, because she had intended to end the marriage. The point of this anecdote is not, of course, that the genetic counselor is also expected to be a marriage counselor, but rather that the best genetic counseling takes place in an atmosphere of openness, mutual respect, and understanding. In this case, the discussion incidentally resulted in an improvement in the marriage. The couple have since had a normal child.

The decision to seek medical care also differs in different American subcultures. Zola (1963b) found that the Italians in his study sought medical care when symptoms interfered with their relationships with others; the Irish sought care when their friends and family agreed they should do so; and the Anglo–Saxons when symptoms interfered with physical activities. By asking how the decision to seek genetic counseling was made, the genetic counselor frequently obtains a wealth of information about how individuals make decisions, the structure of counselees' social network, and the importance of different individuals in that network. By focusing on the motivating factors, a counselor can learn much about individuals' major concerns, even if the individuals have not labeled them as major.

It should be stressed that studies on different ethnic responses are cited here not to convey that there is a rigid pattern to ethnic behavior, but to remind genetic conselors that individuals enter genetic counseling with different expectations, concerns, and ways of communicating these concerns. These concerns may not always seem either reasonable or rational to a genetic counselor from a different background.

It is essential for the genetic counselor to learn individuals' frames of reference, so that counselees can be given information in a way that is meaningful to them. Also, it has been found that patients frequently withdraw from medical care when their concerns are not determined and acknowledged (Zola, 1964a).

Doctor–Patient Communication

Because doctor and patient often come from different cultures, and may have different perspectives on disease due to differences in education and training, it is not surprising that communication in a doctor–patient relationship can be difficult to achieve. Although the studies discussed in this section are of doctor–patient communication, the interaction of physician and nonphysician health professionals and individuals seeking genetic counseling is subject to many of the same communication difficulties.

A patient's communication with the doctor is influenced by cultural background and socioeconomic status, if only because individuals with more education frequently have greater knowledge of diseases and understanding of illness (Samora et al., 1962 and Korsch et al, 1968). Not only are those with more education more likely to express their concerns to the doctor (Korsch et al., 1968), but people from lower socioeconomic levels in general are less likely to ask questions when they do not understand (Zola, 1964a).

Many aspects of American life are being questioned and reevaluated today. Among them is the layman's approach to medical care. For example, individuals seeking medical care are increasingly thinking of themselves as consumers, not patients (Reeder, 1972). Reeder further suggests that some of the changes in patients' views may be due to a shift in emphasis from curative to preventive care. In providing preventive care, the "patient" is often not ill and must be convinced that he or she has a need for medical services. Much genetic counseling is, of course, preventive medicine. Not only must individuals seeking genetic counseling be convinced that they need such services, but that the information provided by the counselor is accurate.

Medicine's Changing Emphasis

Medicine is also changing from its previous emphasis on acute disease to one of care for chronic diseases which often cannot be cured and require long-term care or maintenance. As Friedson (1970) notes:

> . . . the simple world of Pasteur (is) being displaced by one in which direct causal relationship between "germ" and disease is being questioned and in which notions like stress come to play mediating if not causal roles. The idea of stress, however, brings to the fore the complicated and obscure psychological and social variables that hithertofore could be treated by the diagnostician as if they did not exist.

Genetic counseling is typical of a new kind of medicine being practiced, in that many genetic diseases are chronic, requiring long-term adjustments on the part of individuals and families with these diseases. Many individuals who seek genetic counseling need help in understanding the social, financial, and psychological burdens of genetic disease. Without such information they cannot make informed reproductive decisions simply because they do not know what they are deciding *about*. For example, a woman who had had no previous experience with genetic disease or any serious illness said: "I think that I'm interested in what really constitutes serious risk. And what comes under that category. What kinds of difficulties come under that category?"

The father of a retarded daughter, who was worried about his child's prognosis and future, took a seemingly harsh stance:

> Might as well be a little bit selfish about it and say you don't want to be supporting her all her life until you die and leave her with nobody to take care of her. I'd rather have her either in fairly good shape or dead.

When this man was told of ways in which he and his wife could provide for their daughter's care after their deaths, he became less anxious about the drain she would be on any future children they might have. He and his wife then expressed less concern about the chance (less than five percent) that future children would be affected. The risk figure had not changed, but this couple's perception of it had, due to information of a sociological nature that the genetic counselor was able to give them.

As genetic counseling has become more medically oriented, it has become subject to some of the changes that have occurred in medicine as a whole, for example, the use of many specialists and team approach (Fraser, 1974, and Kendall, 1971). In addition to specialization, technological developments in medicine have resulted in a greater use of "tests" and a diminished reliance on the individual practitioner's "feel" or personal involvement. Mechanic (1968) has commented:

> Thus, as one increases the efficiency and rationality of medical care in a scientific and organizational sense, he limits flexibility to some extent, and in consequence limits the possibilities for dealing

with the variety of emotional and psychosocial problems that are involved in a significant proportion of the problems the doctor is called upon to deal with.

In genetic counseling, of course, it is not merely the medical and genetic data that shape individuals' decisions; people tend to make decisions, rather, based on their emotional and social perceptions of this data. For this reason, genetic counselors need to be especially aware of trends that might tend to limit discussion and consideration of the nonscientific aspects of disease.

In genetic counseling, much depends on the counselor's ability to determine what people want to know and to be able to explain the facts in terms they can understand. One study of 214 patients and 89 doctors suggests that it can be difficult to gauge a patient's level of information (Pratt et al., 1957). In this study, physicians were asked to indicate how much information their patients should and did have about 10 common diseases. The patients were then asked questions about the diseases. It was found that doctors thought that patients should know 82 percent of the information in question, while patients actually knew only 52 percent. Interestingly, Pratt et al. found that patients rarely asked questions of the doctor or even volunteered information about their own symptoms. However, patients invariably indicated that they would like more information. Generally, doctors were found to tell more to patients who knew more.

These studies indicate that socioeconomic, ethnic, and educational background can influence not only the way in which symptoms are perceived and manifested, but the ways in which physicians evaluate symptoms. To achieve optimal communication, the genetic counselor needs to be aware of differences in ethnic and socioeconomic approaches to illness and physicians, as well as of changes that are occurring within the medical community at the present time. Such an awareness can help the genetic counselor be alert to factors that can act as barriers to communication, on the part of both counselees and genetic counselors.

9 Questions Genetic Counselors Ask

Men naturally desire health and happiness. For some of them, however, perhaps for all, these words have implications that transcend ordinary biological concepts. The kind of health that men desire most is not necessarily a state in which they experience physical vigor and a sense of well-being, not even one giving them a long life. It is, instead, the condition best suited to reach goals that each individual formulates for himself.

R. Dubos, 1959

Question 1 *How can I tell what people really want from genetic counseling?*

When individuals come in for counseling they seldom know fully what is available from genetic counseling or which questions are appropriate to a genetic counseling session. Nevertheless, by asking individuals what they want and expect from genetic counseling, the counselor obtains a starting point from which the issues can be clarified. It is important to remember that many people, as they learn more about the disorder and the options available to them, change what they want and expect from genetic counseling. For example, one mother of a short-statured child expressed how her perception was changing: "I mean he's seemed so healthy and normal, and then to be sitting there and talking like he's dying and like he's really ill. How come he doesn't act it?"

In dynamic genetic counseling sessions, individuals are not penalized for changing their views or their emphases. Instead, the genetic counselor helps the family see and verbalize its changing concerns. One way to keep abreast of what counselees want is for the counselor to ask them frequently. Another is to watch for growing interest in a topic as expressed by an increase in questions or discussion. Often, a counselor profits by summarizing what he or she perceives to be the current major focus or issue, and asking the family if this summary is correct. With some families, a growing list of written questions and concerns is helpful.

Question 2   *Some people are very uncommunicative. They say they have no questions and answer all my questions with a yes or no. How can I encourage them to talk?*

In a medical setting or a new environment, people often feel shy and need time to gain the confidence to speak. Counseling will be more effective if the genetic counselor provides a warm-up time at the beginning of a session. A cup of coffee and small talk in a room furnished with easy chairs instead of an examining table can help people feel more at ease. One father who had been taciturn for much of the intake visit was a fully responsive parent in subsequent visits. During one follow-up visit he explained why: "You told us what was going to happen. We were going to go there and the doctors were going to examine him and everything. I wasn't nervous or anything. I was all ready for it." The genetic counselor can also encourage discussion by asking questions that require more than a single word answer. For example, "How did you? . . ." or "What has it been like for you since? . . ." require more than a yes or no response.

Often very quiet people are grieving and use much energy suppressing their emotions. Sometimes people are helped to talk and grieve openly if the counselor states that he or she thinks they are grieving, and that grief is to be expected at such a time.

Sometimes the disease and its social effects have lowered individuals' self-esteem or have made them angry. They may feel that no matter what the genetic counselor says or does, it will not be enough. In such cases, the genetic counselor may want to jolt people from their passive, accusatory stance by frankly acknowledging that he or she cannot make the problem go away. However, the genetic counselor can state that based on past experience he or she can probably be of service to the couple, but only with their help. One way the couple can help is to respond to the issue at hand. The counselor's acknowledgment that the couple's participation is essential in genetic counseling often does much to raise the couple's self-esteem and to stimulate participation.

Question 3   *How can I keep one member of a family from monopoliz-*
ing the conversation?

One of the genetic counselor's aims is that each member of the family not only speak, but be heard by others. All members of a family can be encouraged to participate if the counselor addresses many of the same questions to them all, such as, "How do you each feel about . . .?" Different individuals can be asked to answer first each time.

Sometimes people who are the second or third to answer a particular question feel they have nothing substantial to add. The counselor can encourage them to express their views by saying, "In what ways do you feel the same?" and then later, "In what ways were you affected differently?" Even if an individual has nothing different to report at that time, the counselor has indicated that different opinions are to be expected.

If one person has spoken at length, the counselor can thank that individual, summarize what has been said, ask if the summary is correct, then say, "And now I want to hear from A." Breaking eye contact with the speaker and focusing on another person can also nonverbally signal that the genetic counselor is ready to hear from another person. If an individual interrupts, the counselor can repeat that he or she would now like to hear from another family member.

Question 4   *How can I learn more about the people I am counseling if*
people act as if I am prying?

Initially, some genetic counselors are reluctant to ask direct questions because they do not want to seem rude or prying. However, few people interpret an expression of interest as prying, especially if the genetic counselor feels that the questions asked are relevant, and can communicate this relevance to the family. A genetic counselor who is concerned about the way a given family might interpret certain questions, can say, "I'll be asking questions today to learn more about you and your problem. By knowing more about you and your particular concerns, I can better help you obtain the information you want. If at any time I ask a question about an area you would rather not discuss, please let me know. I don't want our discussions to make you uncomfortable."

Question 5   *What if I ask a question and the individual does not answer it, but talks about something else?*

In such cases, the question can be asked again in a slightly different form. The person may not have understood the question or the question may have reminded him or her of an important tangential area. After a second attempt with no response, the counselor may silently note that the person did not answer the question and go on to another topic. Or the counselor might say, "I notice that when I asked about . . . , you spoke about other matters. Is this a topic you would rather not discuss?" Open acknowledgment, without blaming, can help individuals become aware of areas they are avoiding. Often fruitful discussion follows. If an individual does *not* wish to discuss a topic with the genetic counselor, the counselor has helped point out an area that might be pursued privately. Or, individuals might want to mull over a topic in private before discussing it with the genetic counselor.

Question 6   *Once people start talking about their feelings and emotions, how can I get them to stop?*

Regardless of the time available for genetic counseling, communication can be hindered if there is not enough opportunity for people to discuss their emotions. People who are expending energy on suppressing emotions cannot give full attention to the information being presented; they often need to see how they "feel" about information and alternatives before they have relevance. People who suppress their emotions are often too numb for new inputs to register; people often gain a greater understanding of their thoughts and feelings by expressing how they feel.

Asking questions such as, "How did you feel about that?" while individuals are relating factual information encourages them to evaluate the emotional impact of each part of the disease history, yet enables the genetic counselor to obtain the history logically and comprehensively.

It is highly unlikely that individuals who express their emotions will be unable to stop. Even if an explosive outburst should occur, the expression of feelings is not usually harmful unless individuals begin to feel that they have damaged their relationship with the genetic counselor or have looked foolish to the genetic counselor. Individuals who are reassured that the genetic counselor sees the outburst as a result of tremendous pressures and anxieties about the genetic disease, and not a personal reaction to the genetic counselor, generally go on to have a productive counseling session.

Often people proclaim their distress loud and long because they feel no one has really heard them. Once they feel that the genetic counselor understands and appreciates their feelings, they are usually ready to move to another topic. The counselor need not agree with or share each feeling. A sympathetic and nonjudgmental acknowledgment of the feeling is sufficient. Sometimes the genetic counselor can do much to relieve individuals' anxiety and guilt about their emotions by commenting on the difficult aspects of the situation that have led to the expression of deep emotions.

The result of joining information and emotion is that the counselor and family come to better understand the social and medical ramifications of the genetic disease *to that family*. Time is not wasted, but saved, since the genetic counselor can then spend more time discussing issues that are relevant to the family.

Question 7 *What can I do when someone cries?*

Comments such as, "It helps to cry. In your place, who wouldn't cry?" help people realize that they need not feel ashamed of their tears. Sometimes the spouse of a person who cries feels embarrassed by the tears and needs to be reassured. For example, one man whose infant had recently died responded to his wife's tears in this manner: "It was quite an emotional blow. But I think we're . . . are you going to cry? I was going to say, I think we're pretty much over it now. And she starts crying." Genetic counselors will be less anxious if they remember that tears are not harmful and rarely last for a long time. They *can* help by allowing the person a time and place to cry and express other emotions without shame.

Question 8 *What can I do when people get angry at me?*

Often people who are angry at the counselor are ashamed and worried about their anger and may not want to acknowledge it openly. In such cases, the genetic counselor can help bring about a discussion of the anger and its origins by saying, "It seems to me that you are angry." If the person denies the anger, the counselor may persist by saying, "When I said . . . I thought you became angry." In other cases, the counselor may realize the individual was not angry, or may not wish to discuss his or her anger just then.

When people are angry, the genetic counselor should focus on *why* anger is present, rather than react defensively or take the anger personally. People who are distressed by the occurrence of a genetic disease in their family or by information given to them by the genetic counselor may lash out at the counselor to get relief.

Anger often follows sad or disappointing news and is directed at the "bearer of bad news." A genetic counselor who has established rapport with a family may want another team member to give the family disappointing information. The original counselor can then help the family work through and come to an understanding of the painful information.

Question 9   *What can I do when family members get angry at each other?*

When family members express anger toward each other, the genetic counselor must work hard to maintain communication between them. One way to facilitate communication is to suggest ground rules for the arguments or disagreements. Among the more useful ground rules are:

1. Each person has a chance to speak his or her piece without interruption.
2. Each person is to speak about his or her view or feeling without disparaging the other.
3. Neither party has to reach agreement with the other, but should attempt to understand how the other has come to think or feel the way he or she does.

   Frequently couples feel a great sense of relief at being able to express their feelings in a "safe" environment with a third person to help keep communication open. It is also important in these cases for the genetic counselor to let people know that when they express anger it is not a negative reflection on them or their family, but an indication of the stressful life situation they are in.

Question 10   *What can I do when spouses disagree?*

In such cases, the genetic counselor is not interested in determining which spouse is more right or more rational than the other, or in helping the couple to cover the fact that they do disagree. (Many couples shy away from acknowledging, even to themselves, that there is a disagreement.) Instead the counselor is concerned with helping each person to state his or her opinion while the other listens. The aim is not for the listener to agree with the speaker, but for each spouse to respect the position of the other. The counselor can follow these steps:

1. Diminish possible embarrassment over a diagreement by pointing out that no two people can always agree.
2. Note that disagreement does not mean one person is right and another is wrong.
3. Encourage each person to speak of his or her thoughts and feelings on the issue.
4. Encourage listening; people can often listen better if the counselor points out that the aim is not for the listener to be convinced, but that the listener gain an understanding and appreciation for the position the other has taken.
5. Ask that spouses communicate with each other directly about the current issue.
6. Discourage remarks about past disagreements or statements such as, "She always. . . ." by asking that individuals be specific in requests about what they do want and not spend genetic counseling time blaming each other.
7. Encourage each spouse to stick to the issue at hand instead of wandering or avoiding issues.
8. Encourage each spouse to draw up a list (mental or written) of the issues involved, including the concerns and reservations of each. Such counseling can be truly effective, as the comments of one counselee illustrate:

> A lot of these visits here have brought out things. We have been able to sound things out with each other in a very safe environment. I come out of it with a lot more understanding of what my wife's needs are and I think she comes out understanding my position a little more. I think I learned a lot about myself in each of these things.

Question 11 *How can I handle my own feelings of insecurity as I counsel? After all, I am not a mental health expert.*

Generally, people who seek genetic counseling are not mentally ill, nor do they come to reexamine their marriage or family life. The genetic counselor needs to be able to explain the inheritance of genetic disease and to be sensitive to social and emotional factors that can block understanding of that information. Many people can develop their skills as facilitators of communication by:

1. Asking open-ended questions so that people can discuss as much or as little as is comfortable at that time;
2. Being direct in their own communication;
3. Being able to nonjudgmentally accept the responses and decisions of individuals being counseled;

4. Looking for issues and diseases which make them uncomfortable—at such times counselors should be aware that their own perceptions and reactions may be biased;
5. Tape-recording interviews and listening for times when the counselor feels uncomfortable—a mental health expert on a consultant basis can give the genetic counselor many important insights and tips;
6. Talking with co-workers about how they would have responded to a particular situation;
7. Remembering that:
   a. developing interviewing skills takes time,
   b. the aim of the genetic counselor is not to solve problems or to find solutions, but to help families find solutions that are most comfortable to them,
   c. often there are no happy endings.

Question 12   *If I feel the family needs more counseling help than I can give, how do I refer them to a mental health expert?*

In making a referral, the genetic counselor first must be clear about what type of help he or she thinks an individual needs (e.g., family counseling to help resolve hostility between the parents). Next the genetic counselor needs to determine whether the individual or couple feel that there is a problem they would like to resolve. If there is, the genetic counselor can say that he or she knows a fine specialist in this area and proceed to describe how the specialist might help the individual or couple. The genetic counselor should have a specific person in mind and have contacted that specialist to make sure that he or she is available.

Referring an individual or family can be difficult. If the genetic counselor and family have established good rapport, the family may be reluctant to part with the counselor. In such cases, joint meetings can be held with the mental health professional and the family until the family feels comfortable meeting with the mental health expert alone. Sometimes if the genetic counselor assures the family that they can continue to see him or her when they need to, their desire for further joint visits will disappear.

Families and individuals sometimes view a visit to a mental health professional as evidence that they are sick or abnormal. By talking with the family about specific areas of concern as well as stressing that they are seeking help for social problems that have arisen from medical, not mental, stresses, the genetic counselor can often help the family feel more comfortable about seeking such help. Some individuals see referral as a sign that they have failed and that they are not strong enough to cope. In such cases, the genetic counselor needs to point out that the referral is being made because of his or her own limits, not because of the failure or limits of the counselees.

Before the genetic counselor can make referrals, he or she must visit marriage and family counselors, psychiatrists, social workers, and psychologists who are comfortable working with individuals and families with genetic problems. Usually, the best referrals are to those people with whom the genetic counselor feels comfortable. However, a range of referrals is necessary since not all people will feel comfortable with the same mental health expert. To ensure that a referral has "taken," the genetic counselor may schedule a visit or telephone call with the individuals after they have had several meetings with the mental health expert.

Question 13   *What can I say when people ask what I would do in a given situation?*

In such cases, people are really unsure about what they should do and are attempting to use the genetic counselor as a guide. The genetic counselor can best help the family by helping them to make their own decisions. They are rarely helped by hearing the counselor's decision. When confronted with such a question, the genetic counselor must be careful not to seem abrupt or rejecting. There is no single "right" solution to the family's problem. Instead, the family being counseled needs to think about and explore what feels best to them. The counselor might say that he or she could make a decision, but it would be one which fits his or her life style. Another genetic counselor might find a different solution more comfortable or correct. The family can then be asked to try on one solution. With the counselor's help, the consequences of that decision to the family can be explored. Sometimes a list of the consequences is helpful, along with the couple's evaluation of how easy or difficult it would be to handle each consequence. In the same fashion, the family may want to "try on" several different solutions. Sometimes a couple will "decide" to take a given course of action, but after living with that decision a while will change their mind. This is what happened to a couple in which the man had Alport's syndrome. In a second follow-up interview with the author (Kelly) about a year after their diagnostic visit, they reported that the wife (Mary) was pregnant.

ALFRED: Now you want to get our rationale? We both feel like guilty children because we spent so much time talking with you about amniocentesis. In the last couple of months, prior to her becoming pregnant . . .

MARY: Prior to trying, we made the decision. . . .

ALFRED: Our feeling, in a nutshell, is that we don't feel that the disease— the renal disease and the other exhibits of Alport's syndrome are, well, I'm trying to find the right terms. We don't feel that they are so severe looking at them 20–25 years in the future, that we really wish to interfere with the natural course of this childbirth.

KELLY: I'm interested in the term you used, that you feel like guilty children.

ALFRED: Well, I say that because when we saw you a few months ago, I thought we had pretty much committed ourselves to amniocentesis, and just interpersonally we had an understanding of what we were doing. And I think a lot has happened in the meantime that you're not aware of.

KELLY: I see. So in other words, if we discuss something a year ago almost, and that's how you feel a year ago, somehow you're supposed to stick by that over the next year!?

MARY: Well, it seems like we've been given all this good information, and everybody's done their best to really enlighten us and to give us alternatives to having a possibly unhealthy child, all of these great things that medical science can do, all these neat things that I was all in favor of. . . . I thought that was really the way to go and I wasn't going to have any boys because there was a possiblity that they might carry the gene. And if they carried the gene they'd exhibit the disease. It was such a perfect solution. And then when it came right down to the nuts and bolts of it, I think part of it is that he doesn't want to give up the idea of having a son, and I'm not sure I do either. There's a little bit of a male ego coming through, I think. But it's like somebody's given you advice and you've accepted it initially and then you say, "Well, their advice wasn't what we really wanted to do anyway." So we have to face them now and say, "Thank you for your advice but no thanks."

ALFRED: I don't look at it that way.

MARY: I do.

ALFRED: No, not really, because I think your advice, your education is still 100% valid.

MARY: Yes, and I think it's been very beneficial. I don't mean to say that we haven't taken it into consideration and learned from it. We just haven't chosen the possible method.

ALFRED: I think what happened with us—and you may find this happening with other patients—is that when patients are exposed to an idea such as amniocentesis, for the first time, in a framework of a disease that we have, it's something that sounds like an alternative that was never present before, and just because it is a fresh approach it's good. It's an alternative that seems positive at the time, and one's tendency is to go with the new suggestion. And I think to some extent that happened with us. Like, "Hey, here's something else we can do! We don't have to make these other decisions. There are other alternatives." And suddenly because it's there, it becomes at the time what seems the right way to go. But you need six months—you need a year! You need two years maybe to really sift all this out, let it fall into perspective with the other alternatives that you have before you can start to really make a choice and be intelligent about it, before you can really know your own feelings about that choice. And I think what's happening is that in the last year a little bit of emotionalism and a little bit of ego is surfacing. When we were sitting in the room before we were being a little intellectual over it.

Question 14   *How can silence be used?*

A short silence can do much to encourage people to continue thinking and talking about the issues being considered. Silence is especially useful when one or more of the people are verbal and quick speakers. Often such people can provide a plausible answer quickly. If the counselor pauses and does not immediately turn to the next person or ask another question, the individual has a chance to think more deeply about the area. People who speak more slowly also benefit from pauses, as they have a greater opportunity to think before they speak.

Question 15   *Sometimes people who seek genetic counseling act as if they were at a party. They are loud, smile brightly, and assure me "everything is just fine," and they have few, if any, questions. Because of the magnitude of their problems, I know they must have more questions. What can I do?*

The reasons for behavior of this type must be examined in each case. Therefore, only very general answers can be given here. Usually, such people are grieving inwardly despite their outward behavior and do not feel comfortable showing this grief to the genetic counselor. Such feelings should be respected.

Sometimes these individuals feel more comfortable talking about their concerns if the genetic counselor spends some time letting the family know that they are handling the situation well, in spite of its obviously difficult nature. Often the genetic counselor will note that individuals are directing the interview away from certain areas. If they aren't necessary to the individuals' understanding, the genetic counselor may decide to skip them. At other times, the genetic counselor might say, ''I notice that we have spent very little time on. . . . This is surely a painful area for you. I want to cover it today because. . . .'' Much then depends on the genetic counselor's reasons for wanting to cover a particular area. Still other people need time and permission from the genetic counselor to express their concerns and feelings. The genetic counselor might say something like, ''We find that many people who have suddenly learned that their child has Down's syndrome often feel anxious and depressed. I want to tell you, so that if you should have these feelings between now and our next visit, you will know that these are quite normal reactions to the sudden surprise you have had.'' In this way, the genetic counselor gives people permission to talk about issues of concern to them, if they feel comfortable doing so. If not, they can be reassured about the normalcy of the feelings they choose not to discuss.

Question 16   *Is it necessary for both members of a couple to be present?*
Usually, once both members of a couple appear for the intake visit, they see that contributions from both are valued and important. They also recognize that their understanding of the situation is increased by receiving information first-hand, as the wife of a man with Ehlers–Danlos syndrome noted:

> If I hadn't heard what the doctors had said, I would have been somewhat distrustful about the way my husband heard it. I mean, it just didn't seem like a serious problem to me at all.

When only one member of a couple arrives for the intake visit, it is often possible for the genetic counselor to convince that person that his or her spouse would benefit from participating in future. Often the absent person will want an intake visit so he or she can also feel prepared for the diagnostic visit. Whenever possible, it is important for the genetic counselor to establish rapport with both members of a couple so that neither feels the counselor favors the other.

Appendix A

Intake and Follow-up Interview Schedules

The following interview schedules are presented to give genetic counselors an outline of many of the areas to be covered during intake and follow-up visits. The list is not meant to be comprehensive. The use of more than one question in a section is intended to more completely define the types of information to be obtained. Possible revisions and extensions are in brackets. It is not suggested that the genetic counselor cover all of these topics with every individual or rigidly follow this order.

Intake Interview   Decision and Procedure

    I. How did you hear about this genetic counseling service (from whom, when)?
What have you heard about it?

    II. What made you decide to set up an appointment?

    III. Did you discuss setting up this appointment with each other before you did it?
What issues did you talk about?
Did you differ in your feelings about setting up an appointment?

    IV. When did you first decide to make an appointment to come here?
How long after you decided to come did you call for an appointment?

    V. Who called? (M.D., husband, wife)

Expectations

    I. How can we help you?

II. What are you hoping will be the result of your visits
here?
What would you like to know?

Genetic History and Reactions

  I. How did you first discover that a problem existed in
your family?
 II. When was that?
III. What were your reactions when you first discovered
that this problem existed in your family?
IV. How have your feelings about this problem changed
from then to now?
 V. What have you since learned about this problem?
    A. The causes?
    B. The severity?
    C. The medical prognosis?
    D. The social and financial ramifications?
    E. What have you learned about your future risks of
       having another affected child? What do you
       really think they are? What risk would you be
       willing to take?
VI. How do you feel about each of the areas discussed in
question V? (To be asked after each section.)
VII. What worries you most about this problem?

Depending on the individual affected, use the questions
under A (self and/or spouse affected), B (child affected), or
C (relative affected).

  A. Self and/or spouse affected
    1. How has your problem affected your life?
       How has your spouse's problem affected your
       life?
    2. Have you talked to friends and relatives about
       the problem? Why?/Why not?
       What have been/would have been their reac-
       tions? How did you feel about their reactions?
    3. How do you think the problem has affected the
       lives of your parents, brothers, sisters, and other
       relatives?
    4. How are you coping (dealing) with any stresses
       of the disease on your life?
       Your spouse's life?

How is each member of your family coping with his/her reactions?

B. Child affected
   1. How has the birth of your child affected each of you?

      How has the child's birth affected his/her brothers, sisters, and other relatives?
   2. How are each of you (the couple) dealing with your reactions to the disease (to a sick child)?
   3. Have you told friends and relatives about the problem? Why?/Why not?

      What have been/would have been their reactions? How did you feel about their reactions?

C. Relative affected
   1. How has your relative's problem affected your life?
   2. How has your relative's problem affected the lives of your parents, brothers, sisters, and other relatives?
   3. How are you coping with your reactions?

      How is each member of your family coping with his/her reactions?

VIII. As you were growing up, was this genetic (or presumed genetic) problem discussed?
   A. In the immediate family?
   B. In the extended family?
   C. With friends?

IX. Have you told friends and relatives you would seek genetic counseling?

   Which ones?

   What were their reactions/would their reactions have been?

Family Background

   I. Pedigree or family history
   II. Social information (e.g., employment, schooling, income, religion)

Evaluation

   I. How long after you called were you given an appointment?

      How did you feel about the wait?
   II. How was your initial telephone contact with us? (Favorable, unfavorable?)

Follow-up Interview   Diagnostic Follow-up

    I. What happened during your diagnostic visit (or during your visit with the specialist)?
        A. Test results
        B. Other new information
        C. New thoughts or insights about the problem.
    II. What were you told about:
        A. Your own, spouse's or present child's diagnosis and prognosis?
        B. The risk of having a future child with a genetic problem?
    III. What parts of the new information do you now understand?
    IV. What parts of the new information are still unclear?
    V. What questions has the new information raised?
    VI. How did you initially feel about the new information?
    VII. How do you now feel about the new information?
    VIII. Have you talked to your family doctor about your visit here?
        What have been his/her reactions? If you haven't talked to him/her, do you plan to do so?
    IX. Have you received a letter with a summary of the counseling information?*
        If not, would you like to receive such a letter?
        If you have received such a letter, what parts most stick in your mind?
        Were there parts that were unclear?

Family Follow-up

    I. What has happened in your family since we last met?
    II. How has each of you been feeling since we last met?
    III. What further discussion has there been in your family about the problem?
        Have you noticed any change in the way you view and discuss the problem?
    IV. What is your current thinking about the problem (decision)?
    V. In planning future children, what would an acceptable risk figure now be? Why?
    VI. Have you discussed your clinic visit with friends and relatives?
        What have been/would have been their reactions?
        How do you feel about their reactions?

*Some genetic counselors send a summary letter after the diagnostic visit, others after the first or subsequent follow-up visit.

VII. How have you been handling your feelings and reactions?

What has been the most helpful?

Evaluation

   I. What are your feelings about your genetic counseling experience as a whole?

  II. What did you like best about the genetic counseling process?

What did you dislike about it?

III. Have you gotten what you had hoped from genetic counseling thus far?

IV. What issues and areas are still unclear?

  V. Do you have any suggestions about how we could improve our services?

Appendix B

Glossary of Genetic Diseases

The aim of this glossary is to remind readers of the pattern of inheritance of each disease and to present several of the distinguishing characteristics of that disease.

Alport syndrome: Dominant; hereditary nephritis with or without deafness; progressive renal deterioration usually causing renal failure in males by the thirties; usually less severe in females

Charcot-Marie-Tooth disease: Can be dominant, recessive, or X-linked; atrophy and weakness of leg and arm muscles

Cleft lip/palate: Polygenic; congenital failure of fusion during embryogenesis to form the upper lip and or palate

Congenital cataract, nuclear total: Usually dominant, more rarely recessive; cataracts cover much or all of lens

Cystic fibrosis: Recessive; affects exocrine glands of body with production of abnormal secretions resulting in high sweat electrolytes, pancreatic insufficiency, chronic pulmonary disease and cirrhosis of liver; death generally occurs by age 20

Diabetes mellitus: Polygenic; metabolic disorder in which sugar is excreted in urine and is elevated in blood

Down's syndrome: Chromosomal; presence of all or part of an extra chromosome 21 (trisomy 21); flattened facial features, hypotonia with tendency to keep mouth open and tongue protruding, and moderate to severe mental retardation

Duchenne's muscular dystrophy: X-linked; progressive wasting of the proximal and later the distal muscles; weakness of the shoulder girdle muscles occurs later as well; onset is usually before age six, a wheelchair is needed by age 12 with death usually occurring by age 20

Early atherosclerosis: Polygenic; deposits of plaques containing cholesterol are formed in large and medium-sized arteries

Ehlers-Danlos syndrome: Dominant; congenital loose-jointedness and hyperelasticity and fragility of the skin; wounds heal leaving scars resembling parchment

Epilepsy, centralopathic: Dominant; in the petit-mal-grand mal type there are disturbances of brain function leading to a slight pause, blinking of eyes, brief stare and then resumption of activity; there may be urinary incontinence; major disturbances involving a sudden loss of consciousness followed by generalized convulsions also occur

Hemophilia A: X-linked; defect in antihemophilic globulin (factor VIII) results in failure of blood to clot normally; hemorrhage into tissues and joints occurs frequently

Hypertension, essential: Probably polygenic; some think it is dominantly inherited; persistently high arterial blood pressure

Huntington's disease (chorea): Dominant; choreic movements (rapid, complex, jerky movements that are involuntary) and mental deterioration; onset is usually between 30 and 40

Icthyosis vulgaris: Dominant; usually noted after three months of age; dry, thick, fissured and leathery skin; sweat glands undeveloped

Juvenile onset diabetes mellitus: Thought to be polygenic or recessive; metabolic disorder with rapid onset; low concentration of blood sugar; insulin needed

Klinefelter syndrome (XXY): Chromosomal; presence of extra X chromosome; small testes; tall stature

Neurofibromatosis: Dominant; presence of café-au-lait spots and cutaneous tumors which may be widespread

Oculocutaneous albinism: Recessive; diminished pigmentation of all skin, hair and eyes; involuntary rapid movements of eyeball; *tyrosinase negative type*—no pigment accumulation or improvement of eyesight with age; *tyrosinase positive type*— gradual accumulation of pigment with age; eyesight may improve with age

Pierre Robin syndrome: Usually sporadic, but appears to be recessive in some families; cleft palate, small jaw, and downward displacement of tongue

Potter's syndrome: Sporadic; absence of kidneys; at birth the skin is dehydrated, face has wide-set eyes, parrot beak nose, receding chin and large low-set ears; multiple malformations may be present; death occurs shortly after birth

Retinitis pigmentosa: Can be dominant, recessive or X-linked; progressive retinal atrophy resulting in loss of vision

Sickle cell disease: Recessive; hemoglobin has sickled shape when little oxygen is available; capillary blockage can occur, resulting in lack of oxygen to body tissues; growth and development may be impaired

Tay-Sachs disease: Recessive; onset in infancy; development is retarded; paralysis and mental deterioration occur, with death by two or three years of age

Tuberous sclerosis: Dominant; tumors on and hardening of brain; epileptic convulsions and mental deterioration may occur

Turner's syndrome (XO): Chromosomal; absence of one of X chromosomes; short stature; undifferentiated gonads; webbing of neck

X-linked hydrocephalus: X-linked; due to congenital narrowing of channel in the midbrain; fluid accumulates producing an enlargement of the head; may result in mental retardation, spasticity of lower extremities, or death

Bibliography

Abril, I. Mexican-American folk beliefs that affect health care. *Arizona Nurse* 28:14–20, 1975.

Ad Hoc Committee on Genetic Counseling. Genetic counseling. *Am. J. Hum. Genet.* 27:240, 1975.

Aguilera, D. C., and Messick, J. M. *Crisis Intervention. Theory and Methodology.* C. V. Mosby Company, St. Louis, 1974.

Anderson, O. W., and Andersen, R. M. Patterns of use of health services, *in* H. Freeman et al. (eds.), *Handbook of Medical Sociology.* Englewood Cliffs, Prentice Hall, pp. 386–406, 1972.

Ariès, P. *Centuries of Childhood: A Social History of Family Life.* Robert Baldick (trans.), New York, Knopf, 1962.

Bard, H., and Dyk, R. B. The psychodynamic significance of beliefs regarding the cause of serious illness. *Psychoanal. Rev.* 43:146–162, 1956.

Birenbaum, A. On managing a courtesy stigma. *J. Health Soc. Behav.* 11:196–206, 1970.

Carr, E. F., and Oppé, T. E. The birth of an abnormal child: Telling the parents, *Lancet,* November 13, pp. 1075–1077, 1971.

Churchill, E. D. The Development of the Hospital *in* Faxon, N.W., ed., *The Hospital in Contemporary Life.* Cambridge, Mass., Harvard University Press, 1949.

Coburn, D., and Pope, C. R. Socioeconomic status and preventive health behaviour. *J. Health Soc. Behav.* 15:67–78, 1974.

Cohen, P. C. The impact of the handicapped child on the family. *Social Casework* 43:137–142, 1962.

de Mause, L., ed. *The History of Childhood,* Harper Torchbooks. New York, Harper & Row, 1974.

Dubos, R. *Mirage of Health, Utopias, Progress, and Biological Change,* New York, Harper & Row, 1959.

Etzioni, A. *Genetic Fix*. New York, Macmillan, 1973.

Fraser, F. C. Genetic counseling. *Am. J. Hum. Genet.* 26:636–659, 1974.

Freeman, H., Levine, S., and Reeder, L. G., eds. *Handbook of Medical Sociology*, Englewood Cliffs, Prentice-Hall, 1972

Freeman, R. D. Review of medicine in special education. The crisis of diagnosis: Need for intervention, *J. Special Education* 5:389–414, 1971.

Freidson, E. *Professional Dominance: The Social Structure of Medical Care*. Chicago, Aldine Publishing Co., 1970.

Geis, H. S. The problem of personal worth in the physically disabled patient. *Rehabilitation Literature* 33:34–39, 1972.

Goffman, E. *Stigma. Notes on the management of spoiled identity*. Englewood Cliffs, Prentice-Hall, 1963.

Goodman, M. E. *The Culture of Childhood: Child's-Eye Views of Society and Culture*. New York, Teacher's College Press, Teachers College, Columbia Univ., 1970.

Graliker, B. V., Parmelee, A. H., and Koch, R. Attitude study of parents of mentally retarded children: II. Initial reactions and concerns of parents to diagnosis of mental retardation. *Pediatrics* 24:819–821, 1959.

Haley, J., and Hoffman, L. *Techniques of Family Therapy*. New York, Basic Books, 1967.

Hammons, H. *Hereditary Counseling: A Symposium Sponsored by the American Eugenics Society*. New York, American Eugenics Society, 1959.

Jaco, E. G., ed. *Patients, Physicians and Illness*. Second Edition. New York, The Free Press, 1972.

Kendall, P. L. Consequences of the trend toward specialization, *in* Coombs, R. H. and Vincent, C. E., eds., *Psychosocial Aspects of Medical Training*. Springfield, Charles C Thomas, Chs. 16 and 17, pp. 449–497, 1971.

Klaus, M. H., and Kennell, J. H. Mothers separated from their newborn infants. *Pediatr. Clin. North Am.* 17:1015–1037, 1970.

Koos, E. L. *The Health of Regionsville: What the People Thought and Did About It*. New York, Columbia University Press, 1954.

Korsch, B. M. Gozzi, E. K., and Francis, V. Gaps in doctor-patient communication. I. Doctor-patient interaction and patient satisfaction. *Pediatrics* 42:855–871, 1968.

Lindemann, E. Symptomatology and management of acute grief. *Am. J. Psychiat.* 101:141–148, 1944.

Lipton, H. L., and Svarstad, B. L. Parental expectations of a multidisciplinary clinic for children with developmental disabilities. *J. Health Soc. Behav.* 15:157–166, 1974.

Lowen, A. *Pleasure: A Creative Approach to Life*. New York, Penguin Books, p. 162, 1970.

Lynch, H. T., *International Directory of Genetic Services*, D. Bergsma, H. T. Lynch, R. J. Thomas, eds., 4th ed., White

Plains, N.Y., The National Foundation—March of Dimes, 1974.

Macgregor, F. C. Social and psychological implications of dento-facial disfigurement. *Angle Orthodontist* 40:231–233, 1970.

Macintyre, M. N. The need for supportive therapy for members of a family with a defective child. Paper presented at a conference on genetic counseling sponsored by NIH, Colorado Springs, Colorado, February 26–27, 1975.

McKusick, V. A. *Mendelian Inheritance in Man. Catalogs of Autosomal Dominant, Autosomal Recessive, and X-linked Phenotypes,* Fourth Edition. Baltimore, The Johns Hopkins University Press, 1975.

Mechanic, D. *Medical Sociology: A Selective View.* New York, The Free Press, p. 131, 1968.

Mechanic, D. The sociology of medicine: Viewpoints and perspectives. *J. Health Hum. Behav.* 7:237–248, 1966, p. 240.

Motulsky, A. G. Family detection of genetic diseases, *in,* L. N. Went, Vermeij-Keers, Chr., and Van Der Linden, A. G. J. M., eds., *Early Diagnosis and Prevention of Genetic Diseases.* Leiden, Leiden University Press, 1975.

Olshansky, S. Chronic sorrow: A response to having a mentally defective child. *Social Casework* 43:191–193, 1962.

Parad, H. J., ed., *Crisis Intervention: Selected Readings.* New York, Family Service Association of America, 1965.

Pellegrino, E. D. Protection of patients' rights and the doctor–patient relationship, Editorial. *Prev. Med.* 4: 398–403, 1975.

Pratt, L., Seligmann, A., and Reader, G. Physicians' views on the level of medical information among patients. *Am. J. Public Health* 47: 1277–1283, 1957.

Reader, G. G., Pratt, L., and Mudd, M. C. What patients expect from their doctors, *Mod. Hosp.* 89: 88–94, 1957.

Reeder, L. G. The patient-client as a consumer: Some observations on the changing professional-client relationship. *J. Health Soc. Behav.* 13: 406–412, 1972.

Samora, J., Saunders, L., and Larson, R. F. Knowledge about specific diseases in four selected samples. *J. Health Hum. Behav.* 3: 176–185, 1962.

San Martino, M. and Newman, M. B. Siblings of retarded children: A population at risk. *Child Psychiatry Hum. Dev.* 4:168–177, 1974.

Satir, V. *Conjoint Family Therapy.* Palo Alto, Calif., Science and Behavior Books, 1967.

Skolnick, A. *The Intimate Environment: Exploring Marriage and the Family.* Boston, Little, Brown and Co., 1973.

Solnit, A. J., and Stark, M. H. Mourning and the birth of a defective child. *Psychoanal. Stud. Child.* 16:523–537, 1961.

Solomons, G., and Menolascino, F. J. Medical counseling of parents of the retarded: The importance of a right start. *Clin. Pediatr.* 7:11–15, 1968.

Sorenson, J. R., Decision making in applied human genetics: Individual and societal perspectives. Paper presented at a symposium "Early Diagnosis of Human Genetic Defects; Scientific and Ethical Considerations," John E. Fogarty International Center, N.I.H., Proc. #6, DHEW Publ. No. NIH 72-25, 1971.

Sorenson, J. R. Factors shaping decision making in applied human genetics. Paper presented at American Sociological Association meeting, New Orleans, August, 1972.

Sorenson, J. R. In *Genetic Counseling,* A Monthly Newsletter, 1(5): 31, 1973.

Stene, J., Fischer, G., Stene, E., Mikkelsen, M., and Petersen, E. Paternal age effect in Down's syndrome. *Ann. Hum. Genet.* 40:299–306, 1977.

Stern, C. *Principles of Human Genetics,* Third Edition. San Francisco, W. H. Freeman and Company, 1973.

Tisza, V. B., and Gumpertz, E. The parents' reaction to the birth and early care of children with cleft palate. *Pediatrics* 30:86–90, 1962.

Wolfensberger, W. Diagnosis diagnosed. *J. Ment. Subnorm.* 11:62–70, 1965.

Zborowski, M. Cultural components in responses to pain. *J. of Social Issues* 8:16–30, 1952.

Zola, I. K. Problems of communication, diagnosis, and patient care: The interplay of patient, physician and clinic organization. *J. Med. Educ.* 38:829–838, 1963a.

Zola, I. K. Sociocultural factors in the seeking of medical care. *Transcultural Psychiatric Research* 4:62–65, 1963b.

Zola, I. K. Illness behavior of the working class: Implications and recommendations, *in* A. Shostak and W. Gomberg, eds., *Blue Collar World: Studies of the American Worker.* Englewood Cliffs, Prentice Hall, pp. 350–361, 1964a.

Zola, I. K. Some effects of assumptions underlying sociomedical research, Read before the National TB Assoc. Conf. on Medical Sociology and Disease Control, Chicago, Illinois, May, 18–19, 1964b.